Shades of Hope

Amy Einhorn Books
Published by G. P. Putnam's Sons
a member of
Penguin Group (USA) Inc.
New York

Shades of Hope

A PROGRAM TO STOP DIETING

AND START LIVING

Tennie McCarty

With a Foreword by Ashley Judd

AMY EINHORN BOOKS
Published by G. P. Putnam's Sons
Publishers Since 1838
Published by the Penguin Group
Penguin Group (USA) Inc., 375 Hudson Street, New York, New York 10014, USA •
Penguin Group (Canada), 90 Eglinton Avenue East, Suite 700, Toronto, Ontario M4P 2Y3,
Canada (a division of Pearson Penguin Canada Inc.) • Penguin Books Ltd, 80 Strand, London WC2R 0RL,
England • Penguin Ireland, 25 St Stephen's Green, Dublin 2, Ireland (a division of Penguin Books Ltd) • Penguin
Group (Australia), 250 Camberwell Road, Camberwell, Victoria 3124, Australia (a division of Pearson Australia
Group Pty Ltd) • Penguin Books India Pvt Ltd, 11 Community Centre, Panchsheel Park, New Delhi–110 017,
India • Penguin Group (NZ), 67 Apollo Drive, Rosedale, North Shore 0632, New Zealand (a division of
Pearson New Zealand Ltd) • Penguin Books (South Africa) (Pty) Ltd, 24 Sturdee Avenue,
Rosebank, Johannesburg 2196, South Africa

Penguin Books Ltd, Registered Offices: 80 Strand, London WC2R 0RL, England

Copyright © 2012 by LYSY, LP
All rights reserved. No part of this book may be reproduced, scanned, or distributed in any
printed or electronic form without permission. Please do not participate in or encourage piracy of
copyrighted materials in violation of the author's rights. Purchase only authorized editions.
Published simultaneously in Canada

"Amy Einhorn Books" and the "ae" logo are registered
trademarks belonging to Penguin Group (USA) Inc.

Addiction graph © 1986 Judi Hollis, *Hope Patient Workbook*
Feelings chart © Pia Mellody
Umbrella chart courtesy Tennie McCarty
Body outline courtesy Tennie McCarty

Library of Congress Cataloging-in-Publication Data

McCarty, Tennie.
Shades of hope : a program to stop dieting and start living / Tennie McCarty ; with a foreword by Ashley Judd.
p.   cm.
ISBN 978-0-399-15806-3
1. Eating disorders—Psychological aspects.   2. Eating disorders—Treatment.   3. Self-care, Health.   I. Title.
RC552.O25M393   2012   2011047680
616.85'26—dc23

Printed in the United States of America
1   3   5   7   9   10   8   6   4   2

Book design by Meighan Cavanaugh

While the author has made every effort to provide accurate telephone numbers and Internet
addresses at the time of publication, neither the publisher nor the author assumes any responsibility
for errors, or for changes that occur after publication. Further, the publisher does not have any control
over and does not assume any responsibility for author or third-party websites or their content.

For Kristi, whose love and dedication
have made this book a reality

Contents

I know
It's hard to be reconciled
Not everything is exactly
The way it ought to be
but please turn around
and step into the future
leave memories behind
enter the land of hope.

—Zbigniew Herbert,
   "A Life"

Author's Note

All names and identifying details of the individuals within this book have been changed to protect the privacy of our valued clients. Tennic McCarty and Shades of Hope are dedicated to maintaining the anonymity of those they treat but hope that their stories may inspire others to find and follow the path of recovery.

In addition, the Shades of Hope meal plan is derived from a number of food plans suggested by various organizations throughout the years, including but not limited to: ACORN Food Dependency Recovery Services, Food Addiction Institute, Glenbeigh Psychiatric Hospital of Tampa, the American Dietetic Association, and the American Heart Association. The plan has been altered significantly to suit the needs of those struggling with food addiction, but Shades of Hope acknowledges and thanks the many pioneers in the dietary and addiction fields.

Anyone considering using this plan should consult with a physician, dietician, or food addiction professional to see if it is individually appropriate. Those using the food plan in a twelve-step fellowship will want to make the decision with a sponsor. This is not the only meal plan out there. The goal to recovery is about finding a plan that works for you, and being honest about your relationship with food and your ability to maintain that plan. Information contained herein is provided as a suggestion only and is not a substitute for professional medical advice.

Foreword

The book you hold in your hands tells the incredible, improbable, yet true tale of a remarkable woman's journey from disempowered victim to empowered survivor, from vulnerable, abused dependent to autonomous, nurturing leader. Tennie McCarty's story has transcended its own shocking origins and evolved into a narrative of resilience, healing, and profound service to others.

I met Tennie on February 2, 2006, in the picturesque village of Buffalo Gap, Texas. I rather didn't know what had hit me; I had planned to attend one day of a family week at Shades of Hope, the powerful treatment center Tennie founded, but after a quick phone call with her, I had suddenly agreed to be there for a full six days. Was it her amazing Texas accent and the authentic colloquialisms with which she spoke, the grandmotherly warmth, the keen intelligence, and the obvious knowledge? Perhaps, I have come to suspect, it was nothing less than God speaking to me through her, for I was unexpectedly on board for what was about to be the adventure of a lifetime.

My first night strolling around Buffalo Gap, wildly unaware that my own life was about to be inexorably changed, I noticed amidst the charming houses, picket fences, well-tended gardens, and massive shade trees, little Dempsey Dumpsters painted with calm scenes such as sunsets and pastoral views. Critical, I thought the crude artistry marred the otherwise visually pleasing street. As the week progressed, the failed attempt at clever quaintness bothered me more. Walking past those painted garbage cans, my mind judged: *Garish! Tacky!*

Eventually, these painted garbage cans became nothing less than a metaphor for my life as it was at that time, a life that was about to be ineffably impacted by the story in this book, and the woman who has lived it. By participating in a family week at Shades of Hope, I began sensing in an electrifying way that Tennie and other recovering people had something I wanted, a way of life to which I had long aspired and for which I had been striving, but which had heretofore been bafflingly out of my reach. Thus, through Tennie's invitation, encouragement, validation, and example, I began my own recovery from the painful experiences and losses of my childhood. Those painted garbage cans, I began to realize, were a lot like me. I worked hard, succeeded admirably, made the best of things. But while I mostly looked good on the outside (like those painted scenes with which I was preoccupied), on the inside, I was holding a lot of really toxic stuff. I had a pile of old rubbish inside, some of it not even mine, deposited there years ago by others. This old stuff was stuck in the container of *me*. It was at Shades of Hope that the lid was taken (and blown!) off, and in that safe place, with expert assistance and unconditional love, empowered with a practical plan of action and tools that really work, I began to sort through the past, leaving much of it altogether behind me, and embarking upon a recovering way of life. Because if there was hope for Tennie McCarty, there was hope for me.

Tennie's life demonstrates that not only is it possible for the scars of abuse to be transformed into assets, but those very hurts may indeed become a deep wellspring of powerful, lifesaving service to others. Because of her sustained commitment over decades to taking responsibility for her own life and recovery, Tennie became an enormously gifted addiction specialist who focuses on experiential work. A pioneer in her field who is highly regarded by her peers, she combines canny knowledge with intuitive genius, welded together by the hard-earned gift of her exquisite empathy. She is brilliant at understanding and working with complex, even intergenerational, family systems, and she helps bring hope and healing into the lives of individuals and families that seem hopeless and beyond aid. Even the most extreme cases don't intimidate her. I have witnessed, in awe, her leading work more powerful than can be described. She helps birth breakthroughs and miracles that change and save lives.

Equal to the might of the dynamic work she guides are Tennie's sense of humor, her delight, and the ease with which she walks in this world. In spite of how dramatic some of what happens at Shades of Hope is, she holds it loosely, and certainly never takes credit for it. In reviewing a family week, or a client's amazing progress, or someone's denial being lifted, Tennie can often be overheard saying, "God does good work."

Yes, indeed. God does good work. Tennie's own life is a beautiful, inspirational example of God at work, and I am grateful every day that God put her in my life.

I suspect that upon reading this book, you, too, will be grateful that you have been introduced to her, and the promise of recovery that inheres in her life story. If it can happen to her . . . it can happen to you. I am living proof of that!

Ashley Judd
Franklin, Tennessee

Introduction

I walk up to our main administrative building at Shades, preparing to greet a new group of clients. Before I enter, I stop to look around at the West Texas sunrise spreading across the early dawn, thinking about these men and women who have so boldly made their way to treatment. They are tired by lives that feel like an endless cycle, engaging in the same behaviors despite the diets or surgeries they have undergone or what resolutions they have made. And I cannot help but remember the day when I, too, surrendered.

It was September 12, 1985. That morning, I stood in my old blue robe looking out our open kitchen window, with the familiar emptiness I woke to each day. I could smell the dew of a warm fall morning. I watched as a bird chirped from one of the large oaks that filled the yard, the early signs of country traffic crawling across the road near our house, and yet despite all these signs of life, I felt removed from them.

At the time, I weighed less than I ever had, having gone through gastric bypass surgery nearly thirteen years before. Long gone were the days when I was a 280-pound woman. But I could still feel the weight of the flesh hanging off my bones, and beneath that, the hunger I simply could not control. Food had consumed me since I was a child. The taste, the smell, the experience of putting something sweet and warm in my mouth would melt me, and that wave of wholeness would pull me into a deep embrace. I had tipped the scales searching for that feeling in food, and when I wasn't eating, I was obsessed by what I could do to lose the weight.

After my surgery, I discovered that as long as I took laxatives, I could eat and not gain weight; it was a revelation. I had found the solution I had been seeking my whole life. Not long after, I went back to college, receiving my counselor's license for drug and alcohol treatment, yet I danced with food like I never had before. Though I was the director of Serenity House, one of the premier drug and alcohol treatment centers in Texas, I was killing myself with food and laxatives.

Over the last twenty-five years, I have watched thousands of men and women walk through the door at Shades just as beaten and terrified as I once was. That doesn't mean that everyone has been a compulsive overeater popping laxatives every day, though I have certainly seen my fair share of that type as well. No, the folks who have come through Shades of Hope do so with a prism of experiences. From severe anorexics to mild overeaters, there have been successful doctors, lawyers, students, housewives, mothers, fathers, daughters, and sons who have all found themselves joined by one common obsession: food.

In healthy portions, eating is as necessary and critical to human existence as air, but overeaters (or undereaters) do not eat for nutritional need; they devour (or starve themselves) to meet their emotional demands. For some, the dependency might be on potato chips, for others shopping or wine, but when they participate in anything past its healthy measure, they form an unhealthy relationship with it. For some people, they will have only a couple of potato chips, someone else might go and buy themselves a pair of shoes every once in a while, and another might have a glass of wine. But other folks will do just about everything to the extreme: eating the whole bag, buying five pairs at once, drinking two bottles alone. They go beyond (or below) the natural and healthy serving size, and, as much as they want to, they don't know how to stop, because the food or the shopping or the booze becomes the most important relationship in their world.

Diabetes, heart disease, obesity—these are the epidemics of our time. They cross all class lines, all genders, all age groups, all sexual preferences, and all ethnicities. Food addiction is color-blind and it is destroying us. Our food is cheap, easy to procure, and we can get it however and whenever we want it. Sadly, on the other side of this predicament, we hold up unrealistic expectations of what we are supposed to look like. We are sold a size two as a vision of normalcy, as opposed to its being a rare and often unhealthy dimension presented by the few.

Folks who either overeat or undereat, anyone who uses food to manage their feelings, live in the vicious cycle of this paradox. They are alternately submitting to food, whether through bingeing or starving, and then beating themselves up for the behavior. We call this process food addiction.

For so many folks with food issues, they think they eat because everyone eats. These are the most dangerous kind of addicts, able to function within the norms and dictates of society, yet behind it all, they engage in an addiction as pervasive and dangerous as any alcoholic drink or drug. They are able to disguise their addiction by the fact that they need food to live, even when it is slowly killing them.

And these folks are not alone. We live in a world of addiction. If you can't just take it or leave it, then you are probably addicted to it. Now, I know you might say, "Well, then, isn't everyone an addict?" No, they are not. I know many people who would not need to pick up this book. If they gain a few pounds, they just cut back a little in their eating, work out a little more, lose the weight, and are done with it. They are not chronically overweight. They are not in debt. They don't struggle with their relationships or desperately try to control the world around them. But for many of us, we refuse to see we're addicted when all the indicators say we are.

Food addicts live on the circuit of support groups and fad diets, participating in the friendly camaraderie that grows when all of your friends are the same size you are. They are always aware of mealtime, snack time, the doughnut shop quickly approaching on the northwest corner as they drive to the office. They are obsessed with food, counting calories in their head, becoming encyclopedias of nutritional value. They have been to Weight Watchers and Jenny Craig, and have been on every diet from Atkins to South Beach. It's not to say that all of those things don't work, because they do. In order to be healthy with food, we must eat healthy, but we must also be able to see how this relationship to food mirrors all of the other relationships in our lives—the way we love, the way we shop, the way we consume. The food addict believes the solution is in the diet, and they represent nearly 75 percent of America.

The multibillion-dollar diet industry feeds off this dependency. Creating a market to respond to the epidemic, the industry well understands that consumers will typically try the next diet, but they will rarely succeed. If they did, no one would buy the next product; they wouldn't buy the next video. The diet industry's business model is predicated on this need for more. It counts on that local doughnut shop to drive folks back to another resolution, another promise that they will do better. This illness—and it is an illness—leads them to conclude that if only they could weigh a certain amount, eat the right way, they would be healed. They would eat less, drink more water, start exercising, committing once again to that ten, twenty, forty pounds that they believe stands between them and joy.

This book is not about a diet. It is not centered on a food plan. We might offer dietary guidelines to help you start eating for physical health instead of emotional comfort, but if you were to skip everything in this book and go straight to that chapter, you probably wouldn't be able to keep to the plan for more than three days. Physical dieting doesn't work. It never has. Because it's not the food that is the problem—it's you.

You might very well balk at this idea. In fact, you're probably wondering right now whether you're really that bad. You might be looking at your life and deciding whether what and how you eat is affecting your happiness, whether the choices you are making are based upon nutritional needs, a little indulgence, or emotional exigencies. And you might be asking yourself whether you are ready to change, to stop the behaviors you know are unhealthy for you, and that stand between life as it is now, and life as it could be.

Because this life, held down by the diets and binges and broken promises, can be transformed into a whole new experience, radiant with the scent of the morning dew and the sound of chirping birds outside your kitchen window. But until you break that relationship with food and stop reaching for the chips, the doughnuts, the second serving, you will always find yourself living life at arm's length.

I know, because by that final September morning in 1985, as I stood there looking out the kitchen window, I was living a life caught between two worlds: one in which I showed up for my work and family, and the other wherein I lived in the dark world of food addiction. Though my husband, RL, and I had raised seven children in a blended family over the years, at that point it was just he and my youngest daughter living in the house. Most nights, after they would go to sleep, I would pull out my secret stash of doughnuts, peanut butter, candy bars, even melted ice cream, from the car. I would stay up the rest of the night eating, taking laxatives, eating, giving myself enemas, and eating. I would go to bed around two or three a.m. and sleep fitfully for two hours until I would get up and do it all again. That was my life. And then that warm September morning, more than twenty-five years ago, I drove to work at Serenity House and one of my counselors changed everything.

Allen had been with us for a few years at that time. Though he had the long hair and New Age style of his California roots—seeming very slick for our west Texan ways—there was one thing Allen did beautifully: He spoke the truth about recovery. And that morning, he held up the same mirror of honesty to me. Before I could even begin my day, he took me aside, sat me down, and, putting his hand on mine, he said, "Tennie, you're a bulimic."

Though I didn't work in the field of eating disorders, and, at the time, the terms *anorexia* and *bulimia* were still new in the public consciousness, I had heard the stories of Karen Carpenter and others, understanding enough to know that I didn't have an eating disorder. I loved to eat; how was that a disorder? I don't even remember whether I responded; I just remember thinking, *He doesn't know what he's talking about.*

But Allen continued. "You've got liver spots and cracks on your face; your hair is falling out. I watch you, Tennie. You'll be in lecture or group and someone will say something that hurts your feelings and you'll call for a break. You'll go down to the candy machine, and then you'll go down to the bathroom and lock the door, and five minutes later you come back to the group with a big smile on and everything is suddenly fine. But you've still got the dark circles under your eyes. And you can't stay at work. You're a bulimic."

I sat there with the same insolence I have seen in so many addicts' eyes. Because as much as I didn't want to live like that anymore, dwelling in self-abuse, I was also terrified to let it go. Food had been my comfort since I was four years old. I weighed 139 pounds by first grade, and 220 by the time I was twelve. It drove every behavior and choice I made. Allen gave me a book called *Fat Is a Family Affair* by Dr. Judi Hollis, asking if I would read it. One of Allen's friends in California was a woman named

Michelle who was a psychologist specializing in food addiction, and was helping Judi Hollis open up a treatment center for eating disorders in Los Angeles.

I finished the book in one night, and over the next few days I took the first tenuous steps to my own recovery. I spoke with Michelle, and though I kept waiting for an obstacle to fall into my path, giving me a good, solid reason not to go to California for treatment, none appeared.

The following Wednesday I boarded a plane and found myself in Los Angeles for my eating disorder. Those next thirty days were the hardest of my life, as I learned what it meant to be skinned of all of my survival techniques, going through a physical withdrawal that would mirror any junkie's—the sugar, caffeine, white flour, and laxatives I had been abusing for decades leaving my body.

I left the treatment center on a sunny Los Angeles morning, and I knew that though I might have another binge in me, I didn't have another withdrawal. On the plane home, I decided I would take what I had learned and share it with others, asking my husband whether he would join me in opening up a treatment center for eating disorders. It didn't take us long to find a location for our center in Buffalo Gap, Texas, not far from our house in Abilene.

Shades of Hope was founded in 1987, and since then, we have treated all varieties of addictions, offering a number of treatment plans to meet each person's needs. We offer a six-day intensive program for people who might be addressing their weight issues for the first time, or for folks who feel they need a push to get back on track. And then, if a client needs additional work, we offer a six-week residential program which can last until the person is ready to return home.

Whether folks are with us for six days or six months, we shift their focus from the number on their scale or the husband at home to the real roots of their issues with food. Once clients arrive, they realize (often disappointedly) three things: We control their food, we determine when and how they engage with the outside world, and we don't stand for any bull. As hard as it may be, we do not allow clients to use their cell phones or computers, and instead, they are given scheduled time periods in which they can make calls. The world is filled with distractions, and for many food addicts, they have lived in those distractions so they didn't have to face themselves or their relationships. But at Shades, they are compelled to confront both.

Everyone eats on the same schedule, they go to exercise class as a group, they do therapy together, and they live with one another. For most folks, they have never had the chance to be so intimate and honest in their lives. And though many times they show up defiant and angry, convinced that they belong anywhere other than the place that wants to help them, slowly we begin to work through all those issues hiding behind the food. Because Shades is not a fat camp, we are not interested in helping people lose weight fast; we are interested in helping them heal.

And over time, they do. They begin to understand that a diet has a goal, a number, and a time frame; recovery is one day at a time, with an eye on forever.

They realize that what cannot be found on their plate is the nourishment of their deepest selves, the places where they feel the hunger they cannot feed. And I understand. I know how food and weight and life are often impossible to separate from one another, and I have been in the place where a new life was offered, and though much of me screamed, *No, don't do it; don't change,* I said, "I'll take it," and I did, accepting a process of recovery as my solution to food addiction.

For hundreds of years, Buffalo Gap had been home to the buffalo migration from the Northwest down through south Texas. Because we are situated between two natural plateaus, our land was formerly home to many Apache and Comanche natives who would hide up in our hills, hunting the great buffalo as they moved through our valley. And to a certain extent, that is what we do today. We are warriors here, teaching our inexperienced and terrified recruits how to stand strong against generations of pain and addiction. We show them how to pull back their arrow and bring down the fear that has followed them their whole lives. And together, we learn how to feast: respecting food as the Native Americans once did—using it as sustenance and as a means of survival, not as a substitute for living.

Today, my relationship to food is a powerful mirror for everything else in my life. If I'm not willing to look honestly at its reflection, I will always be tempted by the false and empty comfort offered by the chocolate cake or plate of enchiladas. There is a better way. If you are willing to trust the process, setting aside what you know about food and your relationships with others, and if you become open to a new experience in hope and in your own capability for change, then, when that new life is offered, you will also be able to say, "I'll take it."

PART ONE

Admission

To cheat oneself out of love is the most terrible deception; it is an eternal loss for which there is no reparation, either in time or in eternity.

—Søren Kierkegaard, philosopher

ONE

_{∾⊙⑥⊙∾}

Filling the Void

S helly sat in our lecture room, her legs crossed at the ankles, her upper thigh bouncing as we discussed what it means to be a food addict. From Florida, Shelly grew up in a family of preachers, believing that as long as she was a good girl on the outside, it didn't matter what she felt like within. She spoke only kind words, never broke the rules, and had been a good mother to her children. She showed up at all the church functions, believing that wanting anything more than her already harmonious life would be tasteless, if not downright ungrateful. But all the bake sales in the world couldn't stop the voice inside her begging, crying out for more. With a short blond haircut, wearing a prim sundress with daisies on it, Shelly was thirty-eight years old at the time. She weighed more than three hundred pounds, and she was exhausted by it.

I looked over to her, knowing she was hoping and praying that I didn't notice her presence.

"Shelly, what does food mean to you?" I asked, forcing her into the conversation.

"I don't know." She shrugged. "It's food; it's just there."

"But why do you eat it? What does it do for you?"

She tried not to show her emotions, staying cool under fire. "Because I'm hungry."

"Is that why you are already battling arthritis? Why your joints hurt so badly you've been hospitalized? Because you're hungry?" Shelly looked away as I asked her, "Have you ever eaten a horse apple?"

"What's that?"

"You've seen them all over Shades; they're those big, green, rough-looking fruits. You take one look at them and you know they're not edible. You can hold them and smell them and there is nothing that says, 'Eat me,' about them."

"Yeah, I've seen them."

"God designed them that way. The same way he designed other foods to be attractive, to make us want to eat them. We are guided toward nutrition because we need it to live, and guided away from the horse apple because it will only make us sick. But you keep eating that apple, participating in behaviors that are putting you in the hospital, making you an old lady before your time."

Shelly stared down at the nail polish on her hand as I asked again, "What are you getting out of it?"

Finally, she replied, "When I eat, I feel like somehow I've won; I've gotten away with it."

"There you go; stay with that: What are you getting away with?"

"I don't know. With being myself? I just always have felt like I'm not enough. My father was always so . . ." She paused. ". . . demanding. We had to do whatever he said, but I've just always felt like there was something missing; something in me didn't feel right, and when I ate, when I could eat whatever I wanted without anybody knowing, I felt better. I felt free."

I felt free. I felt whole. I felt okay. For so many folks who struggle with food, they all say they same thing: that it's not until they feel full that they can feel fulfilled. Whether through an abusive childhood or just by the pains of life, they experience this hole in the soul—a deep and resounding emptiness that they try to fill with other things. Food, love, clothes, shoes, gambling, other people, are all sought in the attempt to get rid of that emptiness. The irony is that those things only numb them all the more. And whether they are eating to cover up that pain, their anger, or depression, or shopping to distract themselves from the effects of abuse suffered in childhood or their guilt over choices they have made, they are also covering up all that is real and whole inside themselves.

Instead of filling that hole in the soul, they ignore the most divine part of their beings: that authentic person living deep within. This is the child who was abandoned by his mother. It is the woman who never had the chance to be herself, or the man whose dreams were not fulfilled. They know that they are not reaching their potential, but they are trapped by this idea that it is someone else's fault: their mother, their father, the food itself. They blame everything around them, and they fail to look in the mirror.

They hide out of shame, believing that if they were to shine the light on their own truths, they wouldn't be able to bear it. They think the pain would kill them, so they eat the pain away instead. They are unable to see that they were born absolutely perfect, and deserving of all the love and care the world has to offer. Instead, they retreat to these concepts that don't serve them anyway. They think they are a mistake. They play the role of the victim. They don't believe they deserve to get healthy. Divided from their own possibility, they fail to see that powerful, authentic self that wants another chance at this life. They believe that the solution comes in the prescription bottle or the cookie aisle. Terrified of what they have inside, they overlook the solution lying within.

I know now that when I reached for those powdered-sugar doughnuts, it was never about the white coating or the dense cake; I reached for that doughnut because I ached for fulfillment. I could not find pleasure in the world around me, neither in my children's laughter nor in the breeze across my face. Though I wanted to feel them, wanted them to touch that tender place in my heart, nothing could or did like that first bite into doughnut bliss. My self-concept was so distorted, I couldn't be present to myself or anyone else. Not everyone is as sick as I was, but the one thing I do see—from the woman looking to lose forty pounds to the man who needs to lose four hundred—is that our addiction is not defined by how much or little we eat, but rather by how we feel about ourselves.

The Triplets of Addiction

Addiction is a terrifying word. For many, it paints the picture of drug addicts pandering on the street, or an alcoholic in his cups, certainly not happy and successful men and women who pay their bills and take care of their responsibilities. I know that when I heard the word *addict* applied to myself, I was furious. I worked with addicts—often of the bleakest variety: folks for whom the everyday comforts of life had long been passed up for the bottle or the pipe. I saw and very much understood how addiction can take otherwise lovely, precious human beings and morph them into monstrous, pitiful versions of themselves, and I didn't see how that could be me.

When I got to treatment, and the counselors tried to tell me that I was addicted to food and laxatives, I almost left. But there was something inside me that whispered, however quietly, *They might be right.*

My whole life I had been taunted by the words, "Do you have to eat so much?" "You would have such a pretty face if you would just lose the weight." "Why can't you stop?" "I know a great diet you should try." "Stop the insanity." "You're so weak." "It's just food."

But it wasn't "just food." It's never just food. Food filled me from the deepest part of my soul, allowing me the peace and serenity I assumed others lived in effortlessly. Some food addicts might indulge only here and there, while others are physically and mentally impaired by their relationship with food. But for all of us who struggle in that relationship, at some point we begin to lose control over what we do and do not put in our bodies. We end up participating in the dance of addiction. We take the first bite and we can't stop. We start the diet and find ourselves back to the same old habits within the week. As much as we don't want to, we just can't stop.

The compulsive overeater stands at her daughter's birthday party, cleaning up as children run across the backyard, her husband talking with friends by the barbecue. She picks up the cake and walks it into the kitchen, telling herself that she is just going to clean up. She puts the cake down on the countertop and looks outside to see her friends move toward the leftovers, preparing to help. Though she knows they will be coming into the kitchen soon, there is no amount of willpower that can stop her as she picks up the fork and digs in. She feels the cake in her mouth, the sugar melting, and the frosting on her lips. She can hear the children playing outside and it all slows down: The stress of the birthday party, the neighbor's kid throwing a tantrum, life itself dissipates as the fork goes back into the cake and she reaches again for rapture. It is this loss of control that defines addiction. It is not about the consequences, nor the frequency with which the addict partakes in the substance, but rather the cycle of desire and shame that surrounds the process. Because once our addict looks down at how much cake she just ate, feeling that physical and emotional turn in her belly, knowing that once again she has hidden away from her friends and family and sought solace in the one thing she promised herself she wouldn't do, she feels the exquisite sting of shame. She breathes in deep, throws the fork into the sink, quickly puts away the cake, and tries to pretend that it didn't happen. She tells herself that she'll skip dinner later; she'll make up for it. She'll start the diet tomorrow, and never do this again. The worst part is that she does this all the time.

Most of the people we see at Shades are battling more than just food dependency. Though they might think their problem is rooted only in the cake, as we begin to dig deeper, we find that they are typically facing the triplets of addiction: sex and love, spending and shopping, and that unhealthy relationship with food.

Codependency-R-Us

The Buddhist writer Thich Nhat Hanh writes, "The most precious gift you can give to the one you love is your true presence." Unfortunately, codependency is when we lose ourselves to the power of relationships, forgoing our own identity and needs in order to take care of others. And in the process, we remove ourselves from the present that is so key to love. We give everything away that we wish we could get.

Food addicts are often also codependents, having perfected the act of pretending that there is nothing wrong. They're all smiles, working out of their most passive characteristics, always asking, "Can I help you, please? What can I do for you?" That is, until you put them on a food plan, and then, my God, someone bar the door. They have all been too nice for too long, thinking that they were being proper or polite when really they were just refusing to be present.

I explain this concept to a new group of clients. They have just come in for our six-day intensive program. They are all looking for the answers to their weight problem, their struggles with food, and are confused about why I am suddenly talking about their relationships. As soon as the word *codependency* leaves my mouth, a hand shoots up.

Tanya, a woman close to my age with an array of diamonds on her hand, responds, "I've been married to my husband for over forty years. He is my best friend; we depend on each other but we're not codependent. I hate that word. So don't try to tell me that we don't have a good relationship."

If only I had a nickel for every time that was the reaction I received to the word *codependency*.

"I'm not trying to tell you anything about your relationship," I replied. "I don't know too much about it yet, but you have just told us something. We don't hate things for nothing. Why do you 'hate' the word *codependency*?"

She rolled her eyes as though it were a chore just to recall the memory. "I went to a therapist a few years back, you know, because of the weight, and when I told her that it was hard for me to stop overeating because I ate with my husband, she told me I was codependent. So I left."

"And did you stop eating whatever your husband was eating?"

"No, that's not the problem. The problem is me."

I nodded. "Yes, it is. You see, Tanya, coupleship is one of the most important elements of the human experience. We were meant to find a partner with whom to grow and build homes and families, but you can't give and give and give thinking you're going to receive something back. Why do you like to eat what your husband eats?"

"It's easy."

"And that's just an easy answer. When you two are presumably sitting down, having a meal, and he wants . . . what, macaroni and cheese, a hamburger, sweets, do you eat sweets together?"

"We have always loved sharing ice cream—sometimes we don't even put it in separate bowls; we just eat it together out of the tub."

"So you create intimacy through it. You share something."

She hesitated. "Well, yes, but we—"

"How often does your husband hold you?"

Tanya stopped, suddenly at a loss for words.

"This is why we call it codependency. Because you are seeking that comfort of intimacy through your relationship, but you're not getting it where you should be. Instead you're sharing ice cream and calling it love."

She looked away, trying to avoid my attention.

"Tanya, stay with me. What are you experiencing right now?"

Tanya kept her eyes on the floor, but then she began to speak, her voice shaking as the emotion came through. "I just feel like this is the relationship I'm in, so I should be happy for it. I feel like I don't deserve more than what Walter offers. At least when we eat together, we feel the same way; we're bonded, but that's the only place in our relationship where that happens."

For so many food addicts, we are either dependent on the love we believe that other person can give us, or we run from it completely, unable to be fully present to the relationship, putting that boundary of food up around us, just as Tanya and her husband Walter were doing. Though we may show up in the superficial ways that our responsibilities demand, we are forever locked in the cycle of hiding from the real pain, joy, and work that are inherent to love.

BRING IN THE FOOD

From the first taste of mother's milk to the childhood excesses of candy stores and ice-cream shops, food addicts know where to find God's natural comfort. It is in the cupboard, the refrigerator, the cookie jar. I grew up in a household of addiction, so no one was paying much attention to what happened to the leftovers, or whether the cookies suddenly went missing. My father was an angry, violent man who, between his job and romancing other women, came home to spread his rage throughout the house. My mother responded by lying, catatonic, on our living room couch, devoting most days to her soap operas, pills, and beer. My sister spent as much time away from home as possible. But I loved being at home. I would lie near my mother and eat candy, watching her shows with her and pretending that I was an adult. She had her beer, I had my sugar, and together we walked the long, sorrowful road of addiction.

By the time I was in my forties, I was consumed by food addiction. I would get up in the morning and drink a whole pot of coffee just to be able to get through my day, to make up for the fact that I had slept only a couple of hours before. I would then get ready and go to work helping other people find recovery. Meeting with the counselors in our office, I would go over treatment plans for our clients, guiding people toward sober and healthy lives. Then I would find a way to slip out of work, making excuses for other places I needed to be. I would get in my car, thinking, *Don't do this; don't do this. Go home or go back to work. Please.* But the pull was too strong.

I would drive to different grocery stores and 7-Elevens, buying laxatives and bags of food, frenzied by my hunt. I would move around, going to different locations and neighboring towns so nobody noticed what I was doing. I would sit in my car—inhaling cheeseburgers, swallowing laxatives, eating French fries, candy bars, powdered-sugar doughnuts— and then everything would calm for a moment. I would forget about what was going on at home or the office and I would feel nothing but an empty bliss.

Food allowed me to detach absolutely from the process of living. Stepping out of my body, out of whatever circumstances I was facing at the time, I could turn myself over to the blur of a sugar-induced high. From childhood, I had wanted that sweet contentment of being a babe in arms, to be swaddled in a warm towel, held by my mother, and to experience the unconditional love that was absent from my own story. When I ate, I finally had it.

And then just like that, it would be gone. As though emerging from a blackout, sitting in the front seat of my car I'd feel nothing but shame at the sea of candy and fast-food wrappers. Quickly pulling down the visor mirror to wipe off the mess I would create around my mouth—ketchup, chocolate, powdered sugar—I would look at myself with utter hatred and disgust, knowing that once again, I had given in to addiction. Filled with food, I couldn't wait to get it out. Though I had been suffering from intense hemorrhoids and fissures for years, I mindlessly consumed an endless stream of laxatives (taking up to 120 a day, developing a callus on my thumb from opening the foil packets), as desperate for the release as I had been for the food. I would rush home before my daughter or husband arrived, and though the process was painful, I would force all the food out of me, telling myself that I was weak and fat, that I deserved to suffer. I would be relieved of the food's burden, and with that release, a new high would come. My stomach would feel flat and my body light, and I would pretend that nothing had happened. I had been lying to myself for so long, I thought that I controlled truth. If I didn't believe something had occurred, then it didn't. I erroneously believed that I was in charge—at work, at home, and over the food that had long lorded it over me.

Food addiction is another way in which we try to exert control over the world. Whether through overeating, purging, or restriction—i.e., starvation—we know what will happen when we eat (or starve), and we know how it will affect those around us. We might not be able to see that manipulation at first, but as we look back on our history, we can identify where food has been the dictator of our lives and behaviors, determining how we acted in relationships, and the choices we made at work and at home. When we are late to pick up our kids at school because we needed just one more snack, when we refuse to make love to our spouse because we don't like how we look, or when we are incapable of playing ball at a picnic with friends or family because we get too out of breath, food has made that decision for us.

Consumption Fever

It was only about three months after I returned home from treatment that I began to see how money and shopping could help me self-soothe. When I was little, shopping was a rare but exhilarating experience, often financed by my mother, who wrote fraudulent checks or shoplifted, teaching me that I could get what I wanted without paying for it.

I remember, years back, being at a pharmacy with an old friend, and as the cashier rang up my purchases, which included enough bathroom sponges, lotions, face washes, and moisturizers to keep all of west Texas clean, she said to me, "Jesus, Tennie, are you a consumer or what?" And I was. I was determined that the solution I had been seeking my whole life might just come in a bottle of shampoo, a bag of cookies, or a new blouse. Cost and necessity meant little against my need to have. For some, bankruptcy takes place when they take on an insecure mortgage or car payment. For me, bankruptcy took place in the women's department of Sears. It had gotten to the point in RL's alcoholism where his bar tab left us little money at the end of the month. Yet one day I saw this dress that I was just determined to have, even if it meant that I had to shoplift. It was a size twenty-six with a dropped waist, in jersey material, and with foam padding. That thing was so bulky, I had to clear out half the diaper bag to make it fit, but the adrenaline was pumping and I felt the same rush I found in food: the lightness, the freedom, the knowledge that I could do anything I wanted and no one could stop me.

But once I got home, I didn't know how I was going to explain a new dress to RL, so I went in the bathroom, cut that dress into a million tiny pieces, and flushed it, batch by batch, down the toilet. Though my mother was able to steal and cheat without a thought, shoplifting only made me more isolated and empty than before.

The same feeling that drove me to eat also drove me to steal. I wanted more, always more, and there was not enough more in the world to fill me. Every time I stole a dress or spent money I didn't have, I felt just as bad as when I ate a full batch of cookies or screamed at RL for getting drunk. I was addicted to things because I was addicted to what they did for me. Years later, I was on *Geraldo* for some work we had done at Shades with a young anorexic woman. As I was waiting in the green-room, I heard that the guests on after our segment were women shoplifters who used their children as distractions. I thought, *Oh, great, I can be on both segments today.*

The Grabby Psyche

My father used to say, "Grab as much as you can as soon as you can get it." West Texas in the 1940s was much like the rest of America—there wasn't a lot out there, and we had to fight for every piece. By the time I came of age, things were easier, both within my own house and throughout the country. We began following fashion trends, people owned their own homes, and the American dream was thriving on burger stands, Coca-Cola, and the biggest car you could buy. It was a great era, and for folks like me, who felt we were missing something within, there were a lot of things on the outside you could consume to make yourself feel better. When I would tear into that Snickers bar, I was being promised more than candy; I was fulfilling the wants of what I call the Grabby Psyche.

The Grabby Psyche tells us that only through the attainment of more will we feel fulfilled. And so I sought more food, more love, and more clothes. Striving for a gratification I had long stopped seeking in others, I found there was no presence in the behavior. I could not stop to feel the moment. Instead, I endlessly rushed forward, swinging from one escape to another so I wouldn't have to think or feel. I found that any thing could temporarily sustain me if I devoured enough or denied myself altogether. I would vacillate between, "Eat it/buy it/love it now, pay for it later and everything will be fine," to, "Don't eat/buy it/love it now, because you don't deserve it, and everything is terrible either way," and it didn't make a difference whether I indulged or not. In the end, I still felt the empty craving for more.

The first time I met Tessa, she was getting out of her black GMC and was masked by a large pair of Chanel sunglasses covering her child-like face. She had everything most women her age would want: a loving husband, a successful career, two healthy children. She was an attractive and outgoing member of her community. By the time Tessa came to us, she was also taking thirty-five laxatives a day and had maxed out nearly every one of her credit cards. She hid both the bulimia and the bills from her husband, and it wasn't until she was hospitalized from dehydration that anyone knew how she had been living.

Once in the hospital, she admitted to her husband why she was so sick . . . and how long she had been sick. She admitted to being a bulimic since ninth grade. Initially, she came in through our six-day intensive program, and right away the complaints began: She hated the food (coming down from sugar, caffeine, and white flour can cause that reaction), she wanted to use her phone (but we have our policy that doesn't allow phones or computers), and she really didn't appreciate that her bags were searched and her well-stocked supply of Dulcolax was confiscated on the first day. But by the end of the six-day intensive program, Tessa had turned the corner as we watch many do in our program. At our last lunch with the group, she told everyone, "I just can't believe I was living life like that and actually calling it living. It wasn't. I was dying. I don't ever want to go back to that."

After the lunch, however, we told Tessa that we thought she should stay for our six-week residential program. Her disorder had been so severe, her behavior so erratic, that we feared that if she returned home to the responsibilities of her life and family, she would quickly find herself in the same cycle as before. The minute we suggested that Tessa really commit to that change, we watched that Grabby Psyche come out. Though Tessa's husband was completely on board with her staying, she was adamant that they couldn't afford it, that her husband couldn't manage the house in her absence. I almost laughed. Despite her obvious shopping addiction, with credit cards soaring well beyond her and her husband's means, Tessa was suddenly worried about the finances.

Finally, her husband drove out to discuss the scenario with Tessa and our staff at Shades. He explained to her that they were fine to pay for treatment and that her mother had already agreed to help out around the house. Hearing this, Tessa got hysterical. She began to accuse her husband of not needing her. She accused us of only wanting her money. Finally, I stopped the whole charade. I knew what she was doing. Tessa was like a mouse squirming in a trap. Her addiction was going through death throes, revolting against the solution that might make it obsolete. I told her, "This isn't about money. This is about the fact that people love you. They believe that you deserve to be healthy. The question is: Do you think you deserve that?"

Tessa couldn't answer. For years she had been dancing as fast as she could to make everyone around her happy, and in the process she had gotten terribly sick. Now that all those people whom she had been dancing for were asking her to stop and get well, she didn't know how to respond. She had all the traits of addiction, but on the outside she had made her life look perfect. If she hadn't gotten physically ill, they may have never known.

The Negative Tape

For most of my life, I believed there was something inherently wrong with me. When I was a child, my parents sent me a message through their neglect and addictions that went straight to my little heart, and that message said I was not good enough for their love. And through the years I took that feeling and built a case against myself. I see this all the time with addicts. Whether the message is caused by one event or incident, or compiled over years of poor parenting or playground taunts, the addict grows up believing that there is something missing. He is like a jigsaw puzzle whose critical piece has slipped between the couch cushions, and as much as he digs and searches and cries for help, he is left with a gaping hole in the self-portrait he's been creating.

Addicts use the messages that they heard from others, echoing what they have experienced at home, at school, in church, to establish the bedrock of their personal development, of who they are to become. As that child grows, passing through adolescence, and into adulthood, he will struggle with anxiety, depression, and low self-esteem as those messages influence every choice and behavior he makes.

For some, the people around them reinforce this negative tape, but I have treated plenty of people who are their own worst judges. They are constantly replaying that tape to themselves—hearing the messages that they are not good enough, not thin enough, and not pretty enough. It tells them they should just go eat or not eat at all, and the vicious cycle continues. For me, the "fat and ugly" song played in my head for years. I told myself I was so fat that it would never change, so why bother? But as soon as I was finished bingeing, or the stolen dress was brought into the house, the tape would start back up, like a phonograph in a horror movie, playing unexpectedly and louder than before.

When our clients first get to Shades, they all relate to this same experience of lacking. We say to them, "You have a hole in your soul," and their eyes flutter with recognition, because though they know the feeling, they never understood its inextricable link to the food. They thought the food was about hunger, and that the rest of it, the heartbreak, this hole in the soul, could be ignored and overcome by creating successful and productive lives. So many people just want to "get over it," but recovery is not about getting over it; it's about getting through it.

Uncovering Your Self-Concept

As we began to work with Shelly, our overeater from Florida who thought she was getting away with being herself by eating, she started reviewing all the messages she had received in her childhood. After a couple of weeks, she was ready to participate in a family sculpt, where we ask other clients to role-play family members in the person's life. We had an older man play her father, and asked her to tell us about some of the messages she had received from him over the years.

Once Shelly began to open up, it was clear where she was getting that negative tape in her head. Even long after she had left the house, gotten married, and had children of her own, her father would call her almost every day and question her. It was less about concern than it was about interrogation. He would start by asking how her children were. How was her daughter doing in school? Her son in sports? And then he would ask Shelly about herself. Was she helping out at the church that weekend? Was she able to stay away from the bake sale or was she eating all the cookies she was making? He suggested she start dressing more "feminine" if she wanted to keep her husband's interest, and would question her about the health of her marriage. This man was absolutely inappropriate with his daughter, placing her under a magnifying glass her whole life, and implying that if only she did what he said, she would deserve his love.

We tried an exercise with Shelly where she held on to one end of a sheet and the man playing her father held on to the other. The "father" character kept repeating these messages to Shelly: "Why did you have to eat that? Have you gained weight? You'll never keep your husband, looking like that." As the struggle over the sheet continued, Shelly kept pulling and pulling; she pulled it so tight, she was practically wound up in it. And that was when she snapped, crying so hard she barely made a sound.

All her life Shelly had been judged by the demands of her father. She fought back by breaking the only rule she knew how—eating. She had been struggling to assume control over this man who was simultaneously determined to control her. It was destroying her health, and even though she had been able to manage her outside—the right demeanor, the right house, and the right friends—she was a shell of a human being within. Shelly ended up staying at Shades for six weeks, finally recognizing that her self-worth is more than a number. It has never been about the size of her dress; nor has it been about her daughter's grades in science. It is about taking the time to nurture herself. When that negative tape starts playing, Shelly knows that it is time to go to an Overeaters Anonymous (OA) meeting, to call a friend or her sponsor in OA. She often jokes that her mind is the most dangerous neighborhood in town, and she does her best not to go in there alone.

Before you move forward, I suggest you go out and buy yourself a nice journal. Keep it in a safe place where you know no one can find or read it. You need to feel absolutely secure in this work so that you might finally have the opportunity to be wholly honest with yourself. Take some time to use this journal. Either in the morning or at night, give yourself a few minutes to breathe, to meditate on the day before or the day just past, and then get comfortable writing down your thoughts connected to that day. As we get used to writing, we find that all sorts of wonderful and scary ideas can come out. If you miss a day, so what? Even a week can be recaptured, but every time you think to pull out your journal, do so.

You will be asked to do a number of writing exercises throughout the course of this book, and I can only hope that you believe in yourself enough to try them. Take the ten or fifteen minutes they demand to uncover the truths you have been eating over, to discard those lies you tell yourself in the mirror, and discover that person you never got the chance to develop—your truest self.

As you look at your own life, describe some of the messages you have received and used to form the foundation of your own self-concept. We all have a vision of who we are: how we are viewed by the world and how we view ourselves. Look into this mirror of your emotional development, take a pen and a piece of paper, and write down some simple statements about this self-perception. This shouldn't take up more than a page, but will reveal to you the messages you have been struggling with. You can finally stop that negative tape you have been holding on to like a sheet, wrapping yourself up to the point where you can't identify where the messaging ends and your real self begins. As you engage with this self-concept, ask yourself the following questions:

- Do you consider yourself valuable? Do you value yourself less than or more than other people? Describe your self-esteem and how you exhibit self-love.
- Are you vulnerable—either too much or not enough? Do you have issues protecting yourself, and do you become resentful at others' behaviors?
- Have you been known for being "bad" or rebellious, or have you been committed to becoming perfect, the good girl or boy in your family or life? How are these behaviors related to and reflected in your spirituality? Does your faith correspond or conflict with them?

- Are you too dependent on other people or are you too independent? Do you fear you are dependent on other things—substances like food, alcohol, drugs, or nicotine? Do you use shopping/spending or relationships to shape your identity?
- Do you consider yourself mature or have you struggled with the idea that you are immature? Do you self-punish over loss of control, believing that by managing your life you prove your maturity? Do you have issues with moderation or intimacy—unsure of how to create whole and healthy boundaries in your life?

After you have finished this self-concept, set it aside. Much later, you will be revisiting it, seeing the ways in which you have changed, and the new behaviors and messages you will be incorporating in your life to honor that new self.

We Are Powerless

We like to say at Shades that if it's not one thing, it's your mother. A baby's whole survival is dependent on the adults around them, and for most, this reliance falls primarily upon our mothers. Beyond comforting and caring, singing and bathing, when the baby is hungry, Mama feeds him. He is powerless over his environment, unable to voice even the simplest request; he must surrender to the idea that those around him will take care of his needs and encourage his growth and development.

From this early age, we equate food with comfort. But for overeaters, food does more than give them temporary pleasure; it soothes that aching heart. Food addicts cry out like that little baby, upset by the messages they have heard and the pain they feel, not knowing how to nurture themselves in a healthy way. When negativity arises, they don't take the five-minute break or the meditative pause that might help them to move through the passing feelings. Instead, they turn to food for instant pleasure and gratification, to fill their stomachs in the hopes of stilling their nerves.

Food is the closest thing to a mother's love, and for me, I believed that whoever controlled the food controlled the love. Even as a child, I was responsible for buying and preparing the food. Since my mother didn't have nourishment for me, I brought it to her. And when I finally made it to treatment, I saw that the hardest thing for me to do was to be served by someone else. I was so convinced that as long as I was in charge, as long as love was coming from me, and I wasn't expecting to receive it from others, I wouldn't be hurt.

As I became a mother myself, I continued to play the director, determining everything from what my family ate to how they dressed, convinced that I could make them appear normal. I didn't actually know what that meant; I'm not sure anybody does. To me, normal was the families you saw on TV, like in *Leave It to Beaver* and *Father Knows Best*. I would watch those old shows and think, *If my family looked like that, we would be okay.* I believed that was what the rest of the world looked like, and I wanted to be a part of that world. I wanted to be like the other kids in school, and then, as an adult, like the other women in church. I just wanted to be "normal."

I see this so often in clients. They don't know what normal is either, but they believe that's what they want to be and are intent on finding it. They grew up in alcoholic homes, or they suffered some kind of abandonment, or, for whatever reason, they go out of their way to assert control. But because this concept of normal is so elusive, they, like me, are forced to make it up. I truly believed that if my children were dressed well and my husband was in the front pew at church, it wouldn't matter what happened behind closed doors.

Today, I see this as a symptom of addiction. This "lookism" is based on the idea that because we can't control what happens on the inside—

our hunger, feelings, and restlessness—we need to look good on the outside. For years, I judged myself by what I thought others' lives looked like, and I was determined that my family would outdo them in every way. In Marion Woodman's *Addiction to Perfection,* she describes this illusion: "Driven to do our best at school, on the job, in our relationships—in every corner of our lives—we try to make ourselves into works of art. Working so hard to create our own perfection we forget that we are human beings. . . . Behind the masks of these successful lives, there lurks disillusionment and terror."

We become human doers, not human beings. We are constantly overmanaging our lives and everyone within them. We are perpetually preparing for the next show, arranging the actors, applying our makeup, and slipping into our costumes, before we go out and playact our lives in front of whatever audience we think is watching. The sad part is, we look out into the crowd and see that no one is there. Everyone is too busy with his or her own schemes and plays to pay any attention to ours. Because behind the expensive window treatments and underneath the vacuumed rug lives a need so uncontrollable, our big performance can be only that: a performance, playacting that we are in control.

This powerlessness is often so subtle we do not see how the choices we make around food affect our lives. As you read through and answer the following questions, see where you have lost control over your behaviors around eating.

Preoccupation—Give specific examples of times when your mind was preoccupied by food or eating when it should have been on the present.

1. _____

_____

_____

2. _____
_____
_____

3. _____
_____
_____

Attempts to Control—Give specific times when you have tried to control your food or eating habits.

1. _____
_____
_____

2. _____
_____
_____

3. _____
_____
_____

Loss of Control—Give specific examples of your inability to predict your behavior once the obsession for food has taken over, e.g., bingeing, restricting, purging.

1. _____
_____

2. _____
_____
_____

3. _____

_____

_____

As you reflect on those examples, recognize where food falls in your priorities. How has being powerless affected your life physically and emotionally? Where have you stopped being able to control your outside behaviors because of your internal impulses? If you have more examples and want to get out another sheet of paper, do so; catalog all the ways in which you have been powerless in your life—over the food, over your image, over the twists and turns that are endemic to living.

Life Under the Umbrella

Eating disorders are an addiction to food. Like any disease—cancer, diabetes, even the common cold—it is not caused by the person who suffers it, but it is that person's responsibility to treat it. Though they might come in various guises, eating disorders all go through an addictive cycle: One participates in the addiction, feels shame and remorse because of it, promises never to do it again, and then, quite often, without much thought or premeditated action, finds oneself returned to the disorder. This is why we treat eating disorders using the twelve-step program. I have yet to find a program that better speaks to and heals the addictive nature than the twelve steps. For many, recovery groups are thought of as a last resort. But when addiction is running your life, how many resorts do you have left?

The twelve steps were developed in 1935 to respond to the plight of alcoholism. But in the last seventy-plus years, therapeutic communities worldwide have seen that they work for all addictions, offering a program that not only helps addicts maintain sober and sound practices around their disorder, but also gives them an emotional and spiritual support system to guide them out of dependency and through recovery.

Addiction is like an umbrella, and we addicts stand under it to shelter ourselves from life. Addictive behaviors can come in two forms: process addiction and substance addiction. With process addiction, folks believe that they can make themselves feel better through shopping, credit cards, sex and love, codependence, work, relationships, or gambling. Likewise, we see the same powerlessness with substances: alcohol/drugs, prescription narcotics, nicotine, and, of course, food.

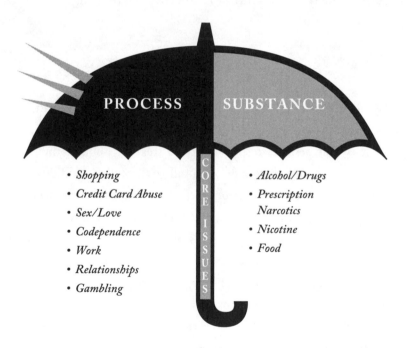

PROCESS

- *Shopping*
- *Credit Card Abuse*
- *Sex/Love*
- *Codependence*
- *Work*
- *Relationships*
- *Gambling*

CORE ISSUES

SUBSTANCE

- *Alcohol/Drugs*
- *Prescription Narcotics*
- *Nicotine*
- *Food*

At the center of this is what we call our core issues—these are the pains and traumas that make us believe there is something wrong with us, and if we don't treat the core pain, that hole in the soul, we will never recover. We will never have the chance to know that authentic self, desperate to come out. Often what happens is that people will come to treatment and begin to heal from one addiction, only to return to an old one or discover a new one. They find themselves tempted by anything that will remove them from their feelings, preventing them from focusing on those old messages, that core pain they have been avoiding their whole lives.

Anyone who uses food as an emotional release lives under this umbrella. When the way we eat is directly proportionate to how we feel, we are creating a disconnect between what is happening outside of us (stress, bad news, unfulfilled expectations) and the emotional processing that should be occurring within. We use our umbrella not as a healthy shield from nature's inevitable storms, but as a barrier against reality itself.

Everyone has his or her own umbrella. As you look over the substances and processes, see where you struggle with addiction. As painful as it might be, it's time to be rigorously honest with yourself and identify the ways in which your own Grabby Psyche tries to fill that void. We will move through the core issues later; for now I would like you to look at those processes and substances and ask, "How do they make me feel?" What feelings are you trying to deny by using them? Anger? Fear? Pain? Loneliness? Shame? Guilt? Joy? Recognize your own umbrella, and ask yourself, "What does this process give me? What does this substance do for me?"

When we run from these seven core feelings—anger, fear, pain, loneliness, shame, guilt, and joy—we remove ourselves from the presence of living. We go from the Technicolor palette of the wonderful and painful experiences that make up humanity, and exchange them for the black-and-white pallor of a muted life. We are human. We were born with feelings just as much as we were born to walk upright and think critically. It is part of our biological makeup and a necessary part of existence. But when we try to hoist that umbrella above our heads, we fail to feel. We substitute eating for living, and we find ourselves terribly removed from the gift of our existence.

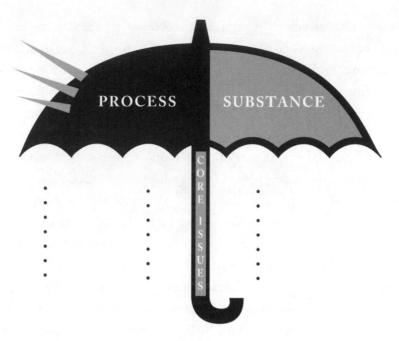

Fill in these aspects of your umbrella—the processes, substances, and feelings that lie behind your core issues. Of those seven core feelings, which ones are you eating to ignore? And what emotions prompt you to eat? Is it the anxiety that you won't receive something you want, or the anxiety that you will lose something you already have? Is it remembered pains from childhood or fear of the future? Is it shame or guilt over something that has happened in your life? Or do you use food because you are lonely and depressed? It is time to lay these feelings bare, to begin the journey into recognizing and embracing their role in the human experience. We must be willing to walk into the void we have been trying to fill, confronting our emotions as logical, psychophysical reactions to the realities of life, and not as the dark shadows we fear to pass through.

TWO

Facing the Problem

W hen I went into treatment, the hardest thing for me to accept was that I had a disease. I knew my issues with food were overwhelming. I had long relied on eating for comfort, only to feel worse after a binge. But when I entered Dr. Hollis's clinic, the diagnosis was clear: Eating disorders are a disease, and I had an eating disorder. Throughout my years at Shades, I have watched thousands of men and women battle this concept. They don't want to have a disease, or even a disorder; they want to spend their hard-earned money to be given a meal plan, and sent home with a pat on the back.

On Judith's first day of the six-day intensive program, she brought her own hand-crocheted pillow to our group therapy, and though we asked that she leave it behind, she brought it again the next day. A relatively healthy sixty-eight-year-old woman with frosted blond highlights and matching denim slacks and jacket, Judith was finding herself bingeing on high-carbohydrate foods late at night: a pot of pasta, half a bag of rice;

leftovers made to last the week would be consumed in one night. She told me that she knew she had a problem, but she just couldn't swallow that it might be a disease. I watched as she picked at the crocheted pillow she had been clutching to her chest, and asked, "Well, how would you define disease?"

Judith works in physical therapy, so she is no stranger to health and wellness. She began to explain, "I think a disease is an infection that through time gets worse, and it can either be fatal or nonfatal, but ultimately must be treated from either the outside or within in order to stop its progression."

"Okay, and how would you describe an eating disorder?"

Judith sat there thinking about it, unable to differentiate between the two, until, at last, she admitted, "I just don't *like* to think of it as a disease."

She's not alone. Whether we want to label it that way or not, the truth is the truth. Eating disorders are a chronic, progressive, and potentially fatal disease that affects the physical, psychological, social, and spiritual areas of a person's life. But here's the upside: They're also treatable. In fact, like most addictions, they are some of the simplest diseases in the world to treat. Does that mean recovery's easy? Fortunately, no. You are closing that umbrella, and are being thrust back into life. If it were easy to recover, it would be too easy to lapse—you must go through the pain of recovery in order to receive the gift. And the process to get there can feel like a roller coaster. Sometimes the best advice I can give folks is, "Hang on; it's going to be a bumpy ride."

The Functioning Addict

In 2009, the National Center for Health Statistics found that 32.7 percent of Americans are overweight, and that more than 34 percent of Americans are obese. This means that someone who is five feet five inches tall becomes overweight at 150 pounds, and obese at 180. When you include that over 6 percent of Americans are morbidly obese, the numbers are fairly clear: Nearly 75 percent of our country is overweight.

By the third day, I had had enough of Judith's crocheted pillow. After being asked again to leave it behind, she refused, clinging to it like the security blanket it was. As we opened up the group session, we went around in the circle stating our names, claims, and feelings. I started the round off, stating my name, my claim (compulsive overeater, bulimic, codependent, adult child of an alcoholic), and feelings (anger and joy), and then I passed to Judith.

For clients, the names part is obviously easy, but the claims, where we self-identify our addictions, claiming our overeating, our bulimia—even our alcoholism or codependency, if the title fits—can be a far more challenging task. As for the feelings, folks are asked to choose from anger, pain, fear, loneliness, shame, guilt, or joy. On the first days, most clients stick with joy (because that's what they've been taught to say) and fear (because they are new and everyone is allowed to be scared when they're new). By the end, however, the person who came in with joy is grabbing for anger and guilt. The person who started with "a little bit of fear" is embracing pain and loneliness.

Judith looked around, squeezing that damn pillow, the terror oozing out of her. "I'm Judith. I don't have any claims, but I do feel joyful."

I paused, biting my tongue at the fact that she chose *joyful* when she looked anything but; then I asked, "What are you really feeling right now, Judith?"

"What?"

"Actually, don't answer that. Give me that pillow."

She held on to it as though she were a child. "It's my pillow."

"I'm not going to do anything with it. I just want you to answer my questions without holding it."

She reluctantly handed it to me as I asked again, "What are you feeling right now? What are you going through at home that brought you here?"

Judith explained that she was nearing retirement, her son was grown, and she and her husband had both been working from home for the last ten years. Though she was by no means obese, she had been battling her weight since her late forties.

She shared, "I was always really thin when I was young. Even when I was raising my son, I was naturally slender, but then when menopause hit, that began to change."

Though Judith's hormones were certainly a part of the weight gain, she admitted that there was also another reason: snacking. "I had never eaten like that before. I had always been healthy. I would eat salads and organic foods, but then it was like I could never get full. At first it was just some healthy treats between meals, but then I started craving sugar and greasy things like potato chips. I was working out and going to yoga, but the weight just kept coming on, and I couldn't stop eating."

She sat there deflated; without her pillow, she had finally allowed the truth to come out. I asked her, "Do you see that by not being able to feel full, that by not being able to stop eating, you have a problem? You don't need to hug your pillow, fearing the choice you made by coming. You're an overeater, Judith. You might still know how and want to be healthy, but if you can't stop on your own—and you wouldn't be here if you could, because no one does this for fun—then you need to ask yourself, 'Is this an addiction?'"

Once we began working through Judith's history, we saw that her eating increased right around the time that she and her husband began working from home. "We were around each other all the time," she explained. "So we began to do this weird thing where we started living separate lives. I would walk the dogs without him. He would get lunch out of the house on his own. We were both there, but I felt so lonely."

Judith is a functioning addict. Instead of confronting the relationship with her husband or recognizing her isolation, she had turned to food. And, over time, the addiction had gotten progressively worse. Judith saw it in her behaviors just as much as she saw it in her weight, both of which prompted her to try and fail at a number of diets before realizing that there was something much deeper going on than a simple craving for snacks.

The next day, she left the pillow behind.

The Nonfunctioning Addict

When Maria walked through the door of Shades of Hope, she weighed over five hundred pounds, and had spent the better part of her last three years in bed. Though she had the saddest pair of pale brown eyes, they were also the most defiant; she didn't want to be at Shades. In her intake interview with our staff, she described herself as plump, and her parents as hysterical for forcing this perceived incarceration upon her. She had been living the life of an aging hermit for so long, she had all but forgotten that she was only forty-two. Her first few weeks were hell for her and everyone who worked with her. She refused food, only to be found stealing from the plates of others, and when we demanded that she attend the morning exercise class, she worked harder than anyone I have ever seen to not move a limb.

I didn't say anything at first, but as we neared her Family Week, I realized that she would waste her family's and everyone else's time if we didn't start seeing some progress in her ability to engage or communicate with us and other clients.

I showed up one morning at the residential house right as everyone was heading off to gym class, and asked that she take a walk with me instead. Maria agreed, and as we walked down a local country road, I shared my story. We stopped to look at some cows that a neighbor keeps, and as they watched us, Maria asked, "Is that what I am?"

I could see the fracture in her defiance, and it broke my heart for all the years she had lived like an animal, caged up in a small room, waiting for her own slaughter. All this time, she had been staring blankly out at all of us as we tried desperately to remind her that she was human. I turned toward her and looked her in the eye. "We were never cows, Maria. We are beautiful, phenomenal women. It's about time you see that."

When Maria's parents came to visit, she finally opened up. She told how she had always hated being overweight as a child, but then when she got to high school, it became crippling. She explained, "The boys would taunt me and say horrible stuff about not being able to have sex with me because I didn't have those parts. I just figured that if I went away, if I hid, it wouldn't matter what I looked like. No one would know and I would be safe."

Maria shared that over her last ten years of near confinement, living off of disability and the confused generosity of her family, she had spent most days eating from morning until night. "I would pay the pizza delivery guys to go to the grocery store and buy me whatever I wanted. I would stock up for days at a time, calling different delivery places so that no one got to know me. I just stayed in that room, eating until I would pass out at night, not feeling or noticing anything. I lived in the TV, in what was happening there, but I didn't live here. Not in this life."

Addiction Is Addiction Is Addiction

Having an addiction means you can't just take it or leave it. The fact is, for most overeaters, they have lost the ability to control their thinking and behaviors around food. Though they may have made great promises to themselves at the end of their last spree, the minute they are standing in front of the deli tray or in the middle of a grocery store, all self-will seems to leave them.

Whether the behavior is about overeating or what we call restricting— i.e., starving oneself in an unhealthy and destructive way—addiction is addiction is addiction. At Shades, we do not treat our overeaters any different from our anorexics. And often our bulimics are either anorexic or overeaters as well. Some binge and purge; others restrict and purge, but no matter what that person is doing with their food, they are addicted to what the behavior does for them. You can call them eating disorders or you can just see them as unhealthy habits around food, but all you're doing is playing with semantics.

If you're getting something out of food other than the basic nutritional needs that your body requires on a daily basis, then you are a food addict. I don't care whether you are eating the entire damn barbecue or if you've had only six saltines today, if you can't stop doing what you're doing with the food, you need to stop lying about how those behaviors are affecting your life.

As you look at the following questions, see how this relationship to food has manifested itself—how it has influenced your relationships, your spirituality, and your emotional and physical well-being. If a disease is an infection that over time gets worse, recognize where yours has progressed. Even if a certain behavior feels like a small thing, put it down; you might be surprised by what a big role it actually plays.

1. How has your loss of control over food affected your emotional life or feelings? Give specific examples.

   a. _____

   _____

   _____

b. _____
_____
_____

c. _____
_____
_____

2. How have your attempts to control food affected your family or social life? Describe how these behaviors have affected specific members of your family, and friends.

a. _____
_____
_____

b. _____
_____
_____

c. _____
_____
_____

3. How has your preoccupation with food affected your spiritual life? Explain whether there has been any spiritual deterioration.

a. _____
_____
_____

b. _____
_____
_____

c. _____
_____
_____

4. How has your relationship with food influenced your work/ school life? Have you lost jobs? Quit schools? How has your performance or attendance been affected?

a. _____

_____

_____

b. _____

_____

_____

c. _____

_____

_____

5. How has your relationship with food been reflected in your character? Give specific examples of how this has altered your generosity, honesty, values, etc. Are you being honest now?

a. _____

_____

_____

b. _____

_____

_____

c. _____

_____

_____

From the following answers, you should be able to identify the effects food has on all your relationships—independent of how much you eat or don't eat, and how much you weigh or don't weigh. It is about finally surrendering to the idea that you have a disease over which you are powerless, and that makes your life unmanageable: accepting that you have a physical addiction to what food does *to* you and a mental obsession with what it does *for* you.

As you read about the following disorders, don't look at the differences. Ignore the parts where you don't relate, and start focusing on where you do. I have yet to meet an anorexic who has never gone on a sugar bender, and I can't remember the last time I worked with an overeater who had never been on a restrictive diet that made him or her feel a little "high." When we play with food, we can find ourselves jumping from any number of sandboxes: We can overeat, we can binge, we can purge, we can restrict, and we can find ourselves with any one of these labels. What we cannot do, if we intend to be healthy, is to think any of them are different from the rest.

FACT: OVEREATERS CRAVE SUGAR

Food is the fuel that helps us to move. On its own, it is an integral and necessary component to the survival of all living creatures. And part of that process includes the consumption and breaking down of sugars for energy. Sugar in itself is not necessarily addictive. It is when we use it beyond its intended purpose that addiction occurs. I know many people who can eat sugar with no problem at all. They will be at a holiday party, have a cookie or two, and five minutes later they won't want another or be thinking about the one they just ate. But some of us are different.

A 2011 study from the Yale Rudd Center for Food Policy & Obesity offered that food addicts have the same response to a chocolate milk shake that a drug addict has to a line of cocaine. The study, published in the *Archives of General Psychiatry,* found that the brains of subjects who scored higher on the food addiction scale exhibited neural activity similar to that seen in drug addicts, with greater activity in brain regions responsible for cravings and less activity in the regions that curb urges.

I always tell my clients that there is a real easy way to see whether you have a physical craving for sugar. If you can eat one cookie without having another, *or obsessing about not having another,* then chances are you're fine. But if the cookie becomes the focus, then you might have yourself a problem. Though sugar addiction is still highly debated in the medical community, there are many doctors who are beginning to agree that sugar can be a physically addictive chemical.

According to researcher Betty Street of the Fairland Institute, "The use of refined sugar can result in carbohydrate use to improve feelings of depression, fatigue, irritability and/or anger." I know that I used sugar for years to improve those feelings. I would use it to feel awake, alive, to be present, and the minute the high went away, I wanted more. Normal people go through an eighteen-minute cycle when they consume sugar. Once they have ingested the sugar, their insulin spikes, which the body uses to keep blood sugar at a constant and safe level. They get that high and then they come down, all within eighteen minutes. But for the sugar addict, that cycle happens even faster. The insulin spikes and drops in fifteen, ten, seven minutes, disturbing that constant and safe balance of our body chemistry, making the comedown not a subtle and easy shift, but rather, a desperate demand for more.

Likewise, carbohydrates also break down into sugar, or saccharides. Though both complex and simple carbohydrates boost insulin in the body, simple carbohydrates like corn or potato chips, candy, sugary drinks, pastries, and white rice can create the illusion of fullness while lacking the nutrients one needs for true sustenance. For carbohydrate and sugar cravers, they become addicted to anything that boosts their insulin, always maintaining and searching for the right amount of the substance in order to create the needed effect. Though they might try to change their habits by eating alone, hiding food, going on low-calorie or fad diets, making promises and resolutions to be better next time, they trap themselves into the addictive cycle of sugar and carbohydrate dependency. And after every binge, they must go through the dramatic physical and emotional crash created by sugar, leaving them more depressed and hopeless than ever, which only sets off another spree to remove those feelings they sought to relieve from the beginning.

A few years back, I had the opportunity to treat a wonderful young man. Jack was funny, intelligent, and had been successful in school and in work, but by the time he came to us, he was virtually a prisoner of his sugar addiction.

As he explained, "Once I entered the workforce, I continued to binge-eat. It made me feel numb. Though my weight continued to increase, leaving me alone and depressed, I would get such an adrenaline rush from the large quantities of sugar, it seemed to make it all worth it. I tried to work with a nutritionist and got on a meal plan, but that only lasted two months. Before long, I was back to going to buffets, eating a lot of food late at night; I couldn't stop. It seemed like every time I tried, I would pick the food back up and I would be worse than ever, getting sick from it, and still I needed the sugar. I was consumed by it as much I was consuming it."

Jack is not alone. Over the years, I have treated so many folks whose relationship with sugar and carbs could mirror the behavior of any addict. It is physical in nature and, according to Betty Street, deadly: "Dying for chocolate isn't just a humorous saying. Keeping insulin levels high over time can be deadly, resulting in weight gain, hyperinsulinemia, high blood pressure and high triglyceride levels."

Though there are many people who can safely eat sugar and process simple carbohydrates, we believe that if you have problems with either of these foods, you should try to abstain from them to see whether there is a physical addiction. If there's withdrawal, there's addiction. When we allow a substance to leave our body, we discover what kind of relationship we have had with it all along.

FACT: PURGERS CRAVE RELEASE

Meredith sat across from me, twisting a tissue into small knots as she described her life before Shades, her curly brown hair hiding her face. A middle-aged woman from Mexico City, Meredith had never been married, spending the last year living in her father's basement, a prisoner of bulimia as well as alcoholism. After a relapse into both addictions, she found herself at rock bottom:

> I got laid off from my job and just continued to spiral down until finally I had to move back in with my father at the age of thirty-eight. At first, I would start off eating normally, but I would be so hungry that I would keep going, and then I would feel desperate and out of control, but the food would give me comfort like a warm blanket. During the binge, I would be enjoying the food but would be angry and disgusted at myself at the same time, until it got to the point where I became uncomfortably full. I didn't want to purge, but I had to do it; I couldn't leave that much in my stomach. I was being so violent against my body, I would go to a different place in the purge, separating from my body, and I would think, Just do it, do it, just get it done. Afterward, I felt in control; I felt safe. I would think, It's okay, I'm back to myself again.

The addictive binge-purge cycle is characterized by compulsive eating followed by the onset of purging via self-induced vomiting, laxative abuse, or diuretics, progressing rapidly from once a week to twenty times a day. Though scientists are still trying to confirm the exact biological cause of bulimia, researchers at Beth Israel Deaconess Medical Center in Boston have concluded that there is a link between the release of serotonin and the binge-purge cycle. Their study showed that after ingestion of a carbohydrate-rich diet, the body converts those sugars, through a multistep process, into tryptophan, which is converted into serotonin, suggesting that the binge behavior of bulimics may be in response to low serotonin levels. The binge gives the bulimic a sense of fullness, and the purge gives her that much-needed release. Over time, bulimics depend progressively more on this cycle in order to get any sense of satiation, increasing the amount they eat, as well as the amount they purge.

As Meredith explains, "Over time, I would repeat the binge-and-purge cycle more and more, spending whole nights in the bathroom. I lived in guilt and then the fear that someone was going to find out, but I couldn't stop. At the beginning of my disease, I would binge and purge once a day, but by the end, I was going through the cycle many times each night, doing and taking whatever I could to make me vomit. My life got so narrow toward the end, and when I finally went into treatment and went through withdrawals, I discovered just how physically addicted I was."

FACT: ANOREXICS CRAVE ENDORPHIN HIGHS

I don't know of a more difficult disorder to treat than anorexia. It is so pervasive, and it can be absolutely fatal. Anorexics are addicted to their own brain chemistry, and they play deadly games with their bodies just to get high.

Signs of anorexia include:

- Obsession with body size
- Alternate periods of starving, then eating, starving, then eating, with starving gradually increasing
- Preoccupation with cooking or preparing food, with the anorexic often fixing elaborate meals for others without actually eating
- Loss of 25 percent of one's body fat

- Occasional (sometimes frequent) purging of food by vomiting, laxative abuse, or diuretics

Over the years, I have watched many anorexics come through Shades of Hope, and have seen them go home healthy and happy people, but the work to get them there is intense and demands the full commitment of client, family, and staff.

Ann rolled into Shades of Hope carrying six pieces of luggage and, until we confiscated her phone, was incessantly texting her teenage daughter, with whom she shared clothes, beauty tips, and, underneath her Saks Fifth Avenue wardrobe, an adolescent body. If you passed her on the street, Ann looked like a normal, slender mother of three, hiding her eating disorder so well that no one could see it, even by her appearance. She finally began to confess some of it to a therapist, who wisely suggested treatment.

Ann decided she would do the six-day intensive program, hoping that it would be enough. She told me later, "I have had an eating disorder since I was thirteen. I didn't know that I had a disease. I used to say that I lost weight because I was stressed, but that wasn't true; I was restricting. If I was controlling food, I wasn't thinking about my feelings, and it made me feel so powerful. I remember thinking how strong I was for not giving in to the food."

Ann had been living so long in the cycle of starvation, and the high produced therein, she didn't even realize what she was doing to herself. Anorexia often begins with chronic dieting, leading the addict to believe that she is just like all her neighbors, bent on losing that extra ten pounds, but then the dieting begins to lead to starvation. Through this progressively increased restricting, the addict's brain begins to release opioids, causing her to become addicted to the "high." According to scientist Mary Ann Marrazzi, PhD, of Wayne State University, "[Anorexics] . . . cause an adaptation to starvation by shutting down function to an essential minimum, thereby conserving energy until the starvation can be corrected." Anorexics become addicted to the point that they are so mentally and physically compromised, they are incapable of seeing their own death sentence.

Emotional Obsession
of the Disease

I don't know a single person who abuses food who doesn't say the same thing: "It made me feel better." However, once the cycle of addiction begins, it is the addictive substance or process that drives all feeling: When you don't have it, you feel bad; and when you do have it, you don't feel good. Like all other addictions, the food addict becomes like a hamster caught in an unstoppable wheel, knowing he wants off, but incapable of getting the cycle to slow long enough for him to safely abort, even when the food has ceased working for him.

At Shades, we are careful not to convince anyone of their addiction. No one but you can say whether you are having a problem with food. But if you cut something out of your diet or way of life—i.e., sugar, shopping, purging, restricting, or even sex—and the withdrawals are apparent, you might have a dependency on that substance or process. In working with clients, we walk them through these symptoms of withdrawal. There are the physical symptoms—feelings of nausea, headaches, light-headedness, tingling sensations in the limbs, and stomachaches—and, even more powerfully, there are the emotional ones. When sugar and simple carbohydrates, such as sucrose, glucose, and lactose, are removed, do you become irritable? Restless? Discontented? Are you angry? Do you cry? Are you unable to sit comfortably in withdrawal?

I know when I went into treatment, though the physical aspects of my withdrawal were painful, perhaps even more eye-opening were my emotions. I was physically sick and emotionally insane. When I finally caught a glimpse of myself in the mirror, I looked like I belonged in a psych ward. Never having gone a day without sugar or some kind of major food consumption, I was irritable and restless, plagued by hot sweats, cold chills, nausea, and headaches, and then the anger came.

It was on my third day that the counseling staff brought the eating-disorder clients to the occupational therapy room, where we were expected to participate in arts and crafts. For many years, treatment centers believed that such activities helped create emotional outlets, but I believe they only distract clients from their core issues. I had spent years driving my mother to and from the state mental hospital, and I remember all the ashtrays and knitted pot holders she would bring home with her from those trips. When they brought me into that room and tried to get me to paint, I equated it with being insane like my mother, and, though I am not proud of this, I proceeded to go crazy. I threw paint cans and markers. I ripped art off the walls and kicked over chairs as a lifetime of anger and rage boiled up in me, spilling out across the occupational therapy room.

This kind of emotional addiction is what makes food such an innocuous substance. Though there might be ties between our emotional state and the depth of our hunger, we are able to disguise the addictive cycle behind regularly scheduled mealtimes and arbitrary snacking. As we see with the following chart, the whole time that addiction cycle is taking place, our feelings are being driven by the food in an increasingly erratic and uncontrollable demand for more.

The centerline illustrates baseline, normal behavior. This is how we feel upon waking—like a newborn baby: no high or low; we are in our most natural state. However, any feeling of "high," or above baseline, will move us above the line, and any feeling of withdrawal or depression will move us below the line.

The vertical lines represent slightly imperceptible changes that occur

PROGRESSION OF ADDICTION

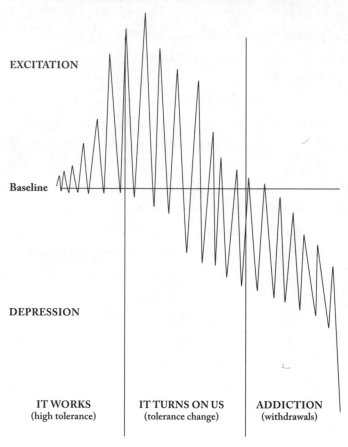

EXCITATION

Baseline

DEPRESSION

IT WORKS	IT TURNS ON US	ADDICTION
(high tolerance)	(tolerance change)	(withdrawals)

in our relationship with food. These changes are totally outside our awareness. They are such slight shifts in how we feel and the reaction we are
having to food that, at first, we aren't even aware of how the food is
changing us. We gradually cross these lines without noticing, but as time
goes on our tolerance changes, our best friend has turned on us, and
we find ourselves living at the bottom of addiction.

Food addicts are similar to alcoholics in that they "didn't ask" to have
this illness. They thought they were just eating like normal people. None
of them went to their high school counselor and when asked, "What

would you like to do with your life?" responded, "I'd like to be a compulsive eater." For most food addicts, they didn't even realize the slow and progressive course they were taking into dependency. Often they find that denial is a much easier route to take than recognizing that their relationship with food has wholly affected their life and behaviors.

It is so easy to say, "Oh, but my problem isn't that bad," or "It's just a phase," and sometimes it is. But if your relationship with food is leading to less happiness in your life, perhaps it's time you took a look at your habits around eating, restricting, and even purging. As you read through the following questions, see where you identify. Where do you do some of these things? If these behaviors look a little different from yours, how? I ask that you try to be open and honest as your evaluate your relationship to food, answering yes or no to the following questions.

- Do you have rituals about eating? Circle all that apply: food lists, calorie guides, diets, and/or patterns about cutting or arranging or fixing food.
- Do you obsess about food?
- Do you hide when you eat or isolate from others in order to eat?
- Do you have unreasonable fear about what the food will do to you?
- Do you constantly worry about what you last ate, and how it might show up on the scale or in your dress size?
- Have you altered your schedule to deal with your weight and/or food problems?
- Do you use eating/not eating to deal with stress, to sleep, to deal with relationships, to handle feelings, and/or to forget pain (circle all that apply)?
- Do you weigh yourself often?
- Do you allow your feelings to be tied to your weight?
- Do you use fasting, dieting, vomiting, compulsive exercise, laxa-

tives, diuretics, stomach staples, diet clubs, body wraps, gastric bubbles, intestinal bypass, diet pills, acupuncture, hypnosis, liquid effects, drugs or alcohol, or restricting to control your food? (circle all that apply)
- Do you have an increasing inability to control how you eat?
- Do you have more frequent thoughts about food? More frequent loss of control with your diets and binges?

Many of us have tried to disguise these behaviors as "normal," brushing them off with the excuse that all men and women think about their weight or struggle with food, but to do so is to ignore reality: These are the classic symptoms of a food addict.

Caging the Tiger

It doesn't matter how you relate to food; whether through the binge-purge, overeating, or restrictive addiction cycle, you battle your disease all the same. Unfortunately, for all folks who struggle with food, they must also face the same set of challenges when they finally try to become healthy. For the alcoholic or the drug addict, he or she is able to lock up the tiger of addiction and throw away the key. But with food it's different. You have to take that tiger out of the cage three times a day. You must train him, walk him around your kitchen, and be able to put him back in the cage without getting yourself mauled.

In the book *Anorexics and Bulimics Anonymous*, by the anonymous fellowship of that twelve-step group, the authors write, "We have a body that cannot deviate in safety from sober eating practices, coupled with a mind that ensures that we cannot stay sober." By sober, they mean engaging in sound and healthy eating habits. At Shades, we call it abstinence. Though many people have different versions of abstinence, the end result is the same: We do not eat foods or participate in behaviors that may trigger our food addiction.

Eating healthy has never been about what you weigh or the calories you count. This is why diets don't work: because we cannot eat with an end result in sight, some number on our scale or those twelve hundred calories dangling like a guillotine over our head. If we do, we are sure to think that once that magic number has been achieved, we have been cured. We will return to our normal habits, believing that now that the weight is off, we won't go back to the worse ends of our eating. When we do this, we are hanging a bloody steak in front of our tiger, singing, "Hey, kitty, kitty," and acting shocked when he attacks.

I want to make this clear: If you are dying of this disease, do not hesitate. Put down this book, call a treatment center near you, and get yourself help today. It is not a matter of trying the latest program or making some easy life fixes; you are battling a disease, and if you fear you are losing, you must get help immediately.

Uncover, Discover, and Discard

Though treatment is good and necessary for many people, I always like to remind folks that recovery is free. There are many wonderful twelve-step programs that can help you, not only with what you put in your mouth, but with what goes on between your ears and in your heart. We can read all the books we want, do the exercise videos, and try the latest diet, but recovery is a daily commitment, which lends itself to a lifetime of joy.

I watch people come into treatment every day. Each of them is different, but the symptoms are the same. They are broken. They are hurting. They are either withdrawn or acting out. They don't want to be in treatment yet know they are all out of options. They have been living in fear their whole lives, and they do not know how to get out. And then they start to detox. Once they get past that—the first week or ten days— they begin to open up, peeling off the first layer that separates them from the world, and you can see the change in them. They will begin that process of uncovering, discovering, and discarding: uncovering the past and the feelings attached to it, discovering their true self, and discarding the old behaviors and ideas that no longer work once they are freed of addiction.

As we move through the work, feel free to use your journal or another notebook for the included exercises. Also, you will need seven different-colored markers or highlighters for some of the work we will be doing.

We are getting ready to make soup here, cleaning and chopping our ingredients, bringing our broth to boil. In the end, it will be a delicious brew that will fulfill and sustain you like no food ever has.

We begin with a *belief* that recovery might work; we make a *decision* that it will work; we take *action* to make it work; and, seeing the *results* of the work, we will receive *faith* in the process.

PART TWO

Belief

From one human being to another everything is so difficult and so unrehearsed and so without a model and example that one would have to live within every relationship with complete attentiveness and be creative in every moment that requires something new and poses tasks and questions and demands.

—RAINER MARIA RILKE

❧❦

THREE

Breaking the Cycle

A s a parent, I wanted my children's lives to look much different from my own. I didn't want to pass along the playbook I had been given by my parents, repeating the fear and addictions that raged throughout my childhood. And though in many ways we did do things differently—the house was always clean; the children were fed; RL, when sober, was far more attentive and patient than my own father—what didn't change were those core beliefs, those hereditary systems of behavior relating to how to respond to life. I had learned that when life gave you lemons, you made lemon pound cake and ate the whole thing; RL added them to his cocktail, and my children learned to do both, as together we raised a family of addicts.

Sadly, we can teach only what was given to us as children, passing along the survival skills that we inherited from our own parents. Without consistent attentiveness and questioning, we are poised to teach this behavioral model—how to react to challenges, process feelings, and engage with others—to the next generation.

For some, this is an absolutely functional course, wherein healthy systems are passed along. But for others, the cycle is burdened by addiction and steeped in unhealthy behaviors. Parents either fail to teach their children proper survival skills, abandon their children altogether, or they are so insane, angry, or unhealthy themselves that they can offer only a belief system filled with unprocessed and distorted feelings. Because the parent was not taught or did not learn how to create a model for emotional balance, they propagate the troubled world philosophy that was taught to them, continuing the cycle until, finally, someone in the family system gets fed up and says, "Forget this—I'm trying something else."

By the time she made it to our six-day intensive program, Cindy had been struggling with her weight for more than thirty years. A high school teacher with short gray hair, she knit sweaters and hummed as she walked, determined to bring cheer to everyone around her. She had spent her life catering to the needs of others: her students, her husband, her parents, and her daughters, but she had never seen that as a problem until she also started responding with rage.

By her second day at Shades, Cindy didn't want to be helping anyone. After three decades of being fueled by sugar and caffeine, Cindy battled immense withdrawals. As we went around in group therapy, everyone sharing how he or she was feeling, Cindy sat there slumped over, clutching her head. Finally, it was Cindy's opportunity to participate. She looked around the room before her head fell back into her hand as she muttered, "I want to die."

"Why do you say that, Cindy? Look up; we're all here for you."

Again, she raised her head just enough to say, "This is wrong what you're doing. We should at least be able to have a cup of coffee."

I understood, explaining, "We can't do what we've always done and expect life to be different. That's why we're all trying to do something new here, because we want to do things differently. Don't you?"

Cindy didn't say anything, pouting at my response.

"Why did you come here?"

Her eyes welled up. "I think I just wanted to get away."

"From what?"

"From my job, my family—my daughters are teenagers now—and I just needed a break."

"A break from the work? Or just from being good all the time?"

She nodded. "It's really exhausting, you know. I feel like I'm either eating because of someone else's behavior, or I'm yelling at them for it. It's like my father used to do. If anything was out of place, he would lose it. And now I do the same thing to my daughters. I won't let things be; nothing can be out of place or I go crazy, and that's not who I am."

She put her head back down in her hands as I asked, "What about you, Cindy? Are you allowed to be out of place?"

She looked up, slowly shaking her head, a sad smile crossing her face. "No. But I feel like it all the time. I've always felt that way."

For so many families, they don't see the demands they place on one another; nor do they question their identities and the roles they have played their whole lives. Human beings are intensely magnificent creations with a perceptual sensitivity that allows us to feel pressure on our fingertips at only .00004 of an inch; we are capable of seeing a burning candle from twenty-eight miles away, and can gauge the direction of a sound's origin based on a .00003-second difference in its arrival from one ear to another. Yet we walk through the emotional landscapes of our lives blind and deaf to what is being asked of us, complying nonetheless.

When families join our clients during Family Week, we try to show them how this transformation might be possible not only for the clients, but for the whole family. You cannot take an addict out of a broken system, help the addict recover, and then return them to the same broken system and expect them to succeed. We show families that they didn't cause their loved one's disorder; they can't cure or control the addiction, but they can contribute to healing it. Either the family joins in that process, or the addict must change his role in the family dynamic, leaving behind the belief system that has echoed through his family for generations.

The Old, Dead Chickens

When I was little, I used to visit my father's mother, Mama Johnson, in Ardmore, Oklahoma. Regardless of the season, her yard was covered in beautiful flowers, with something always in bloom. One day I was playing among the roses and oleanders when I noticed a terrible smell. I heard my grandmother near the chicken coop, and as I tiptoed back there, the stench only increased. Finally I found my grandmother standing in the coop, holding a squawking chicken. Barehanded, she quickly chopped off the bird's head, and then looked up at me and smiled. "This is going to be a nice one."

She dropped the chicken, leaving it to flop on the ground, blood draining out of it and into a dark stain in the dirt. The blood from the previous dead chickens had begun to rot and stink, wafting across her otherwise enchanted garden.

I carried the memory of that dead chicken for years, a dark and threatening reminder that as beautiful as life might sometimes appear, there was always the threat of death or destruction lurking around the corner. My sick parents only furthered this notion by always presenting two fronts: one in which there was love and kindness, and the other mired in violence and abuse. Those dead chickens symbolized my "family baggage."

Figuratively, each one of us fills a tow sack with our rotting chicken carcasses—these stories and philosophies we've been given—convinced that we will starve without them. We throw that bag over our shoulder and proceed to carry it through life's journey, no matter how heavy or putrid, and we fear that if we were to put it down, we would have nothing left to define us.

Most of us go through life thinking that if we could find someone else to carry this great weight, it wouldn't be so burdensome. And so we look for a spouse who might help, unaware that anyone who would be attracted to someone carrying a big, fat bag of dead chickens probably has his or her own weight to tow. Like water, sickness seeks its own level. We are able to connect only with people whose belief systems echo our own, whose language either sounds like the healthy messaging we received as children, or the broken record of the dysfunctional cycle in which so many of us were raised. We will carry these bags for decades, passing them on to other generations, resentful that the partners we have chosen fail to recognize the weight we carry or offer to help us carry it.

Cindy finally admitted to being raised by an alcoholic father and a terrified and passive mother. She married her husband, Chris, moving away from her family with the hopes of a new life. And though over the years they built a nice house in Wisconsin, with a three-car garage and a big porch nestled into the edge of a wooded area, she found herself reliving her childhood. Not far into their marriage, Cindy realized she had wed an alcoholic, and though over the years Chris's drinking waxed and waned, she grew into the terrified and passive wife she had always resented her mother for being. She shared with me on her third day of treatment, "I didn't want to marry my father. I left my hometown so that wouldn't be my fate, but I brought it all with me. I was running from something; I always knew that, but it seemed like wherever I ran, there it was. I am afraid I might be running from me."

As we began to do the work, Cindy realized that it was hard to run from someone she had never met, because throughout her childhood and marriage, she had never had the opportunity to be herself:

> It was like I was a slave to my household, taking care of everyone. I felt like I was always dragging the family out of bed, dragging them to church, dragging them through life. I needed energy to keep pulling these people behind me, and that's why I ate. How else was I going to get through the day if not by eating? Finally, I just got so tired, I couldn't do it anymore; even the food exhausted me. I wanted to go to bed, to fall asleep and never wake up.

Her whole life, Cindy had been shaped by other people's addictions. She had tried to do right by her father, mother, husband, and children, defined by the belief system she'd internalized. She had been taught that her lot was suffering, her role martyrdom, and so she ate her way through the pain caused by this conviction. Until finally her choice was simple: either be broken by her old role or learn to find a new one.

Sick as Our Secrets

Many addicts have lived either in their heads or their hearts, feeling everything or nothing at all, incapable of connecting their intellectual understanding of their behaviors and the emotional impulses that drive them. There are only eighteen inches between the head and the heart, the distance between our hand and elbow, yet despite this short path, our emotions and intellect can be blocked from each other. In between them stands a lifetime of secrets and unrecognized patterns, often held in check by the family who has instilled them.

We are only as sick as our secrets, and unfortunately, the family dynamic is built on those secrets. In order to recover from addiction of any type, addicts must be willing to open the door to honesty, not only for themselves, but also for their parents, guardians, spouse, siblings, and children. It is an opportunity for everyone to uncover, discover, and discard the painful family legacies and dysfunctional dynamics that they have been convinced are normal.

Ten years ago, Katherine found her way to Shades after a decades-long struggle with bulimia. She was in her midthirties and the daughter of a prominent businessman in Chicago who employed nearly everyone in the family, including Katherine, her siblings, even her husband. Her older brother had begun to take over the family fortune and business, putting him in power over Katherine and the other siblings.

Unfortunately for Katherine, her disease was so tied up in the relationship with her family that it was hard for her to see one from the other. She knew she was sick and getting sicker, but she had long disconnected from the idea that the family dynamic in which she was raised controlled her emotions. Sadly, nothing could be further from the truth—she was a puppet to their whims, their dysfunctions, always being pulled in whatever direction her father and older brother insisted upon. After our staff worked with her for a couple of weeks, Katherine finally confessed the secret she had been holding her whole life: From the age of twelve to thirteen that older brother, who had recently become Katherine's boss, had sexually molested her. She had told only one psychiatrist with whom she had worked a number of years before. When that psychiatrist recommended that Katherine come forward with the allegations, she stopped seeing the doctor and never told anyone again. But by the time she came to us, she was so sick she couldn't hold it in any longer. She explained to me later:

My brother would abuse me one night and then the next day act as though nothing had happened. And so I grew up with all these strange body issues; I hated for anyone to touch me. I just wanted to eat so it would all go away. I have a lot of guilt about finally sharing what happened, that whole thing of telling the secret, but I knew it was the right thing to do. I couldn't have held it in any longer.

After Katherine came forth with the allegations, there was a lot of pain and divisiveness in her family to work through, but her husband stood by her side. They left the family business and started out on their own, finally free from the emotional and financial shackles that had bound Katherine to her pain and illness for more than twenty years. Katherine had always feared having children because of what happened to her, but after a few years of intense therapy, she felt she was ready. Last year, she and her husband welcomed a daughter. She told me at that time, "I found out that until you learn to love yourself, you really can't love other people—or your life. Today I know the truth; I know my truth. And I have created a new family because of it."

Food addicts live in that heart of darkness that secrets create, unable to see the light, trapped by these pains and traumas of their childhood. As much as we try to hide them behind our children and parents, mask them with food and shopping, anchor them with marriage and compliant cheer, our secrets will always come back. They are there to remind us that we will continue to be sick until we are willing to confront them.

IDENTIFYING YOUR FAMILY'S VALUES

A major part of identifying our family dynamic is to recognize what messages our parents offered us—what did we learn about being healthy, resourceful individuals in this world? In order to do so, take out some paper and write a letter to both your mother and father, detailing all the messages you heard in childhood, disclosing those secrets that you were taught to keep. Identify some of the dead chickens that were passed along to you—those outdated messages about how to be and belong in the world. Tell your parents how they made you feel—physically, emotionally, and spiritually. What were you told about your body? What were the roles of food and body image in your upbringing? How was touch used in your household? Describe what the emotional environment was like. Did you feel loved? Did your parents expect you to think or feel in certain ways? How were emotions handled in the household? What was the spiritual dynamic? Was there an intimacy between you and your parents? Was there intimacy between them? Did you trust them and did you feel trusted?

As you write each of these letters, try to write them with both hands—your dominant (for many people, this would be the right hand) and nondominant hand. Studies have shown that when we use our dominant hand, only the dominant part of the brain is activated; when we use the nondominant, both parts are, forcing us to do something different, from which the results can be quite telling. After you have spent some time recalling those relationships, set the letters aside. You will not be sending these letters. They are yours to keep and learn from, to see where and how your belief systems were formed. We will use them again later in the book, but as you move through the various exercises, feel free to pull them out. Use them as a foundation, a guide to those early messages that you were offered in childhood.

Denial—Don't. Even. Know. I. Am. Lying.

I met RL in a tornado cellar, so it's no wonder our relationship was mired in dark secrets and the dirty old cobwebs of denial. I was eight and it was tornado season in west Texas, which sent us all running one afternoon to the only available basement in our community. Shoved into the dark room amid strangers and neighbors, I found myself on the lap of a young man. I remember I felt terribly embarrassed. I hated my weight and was convinced I was hurting the long, bony thighs of the man underneath me. I didn't even turn to look at him, waiting patiently for the storm to pass before I could escape. Later, RL's mother would tell me that young man was actually my future husband, but I was too afraid to have even glimpsed his face.

After we married, RL and I raised our children in that same darkness, storing away our secrets like jars of pickles and peaches. I dressed up the basement of our addictions, painting windows on its walls to make it look like a beautiful home. I stressed all day long about what we looked like, what I weighed, whether RL would come home sober that night, or whether anyone had found the empty jar of peanut butter I had devoured the night before. Then I put on my smile, strapping that grin to my face, and pretended that we were all living in the light. I was dying of a disease that I didn't know existed, and I didn't even know I was lying.

Denial ran so deep and for so long in my story that even as I entered Al-Anon, and later participated in RL's recovery program, I did not see that I, too, lived in addiction. I was like one of those terrible preachers who expounds against adultery all while sleeping with his wife's sister. I was behaving like an acolyte of the recovery movement, talking emphatically about its power to heal, before heading home to eat myself sick. But once that terrible mirror was held up, once the light slipped through the small crack of my denial, it became clear that I could no longer hide nor lie about my behaviors. And then I went into recovery myself and I knew that the old ways of being were no longer going to work. I began to get honest, and I wanted the same from others—my mother, my father, RL, and my children. And it wasn't always easy. The tornado of truth had touched down, ripping off the roof and tearing open the well-crafted lies on which we'd built our lives.

But once I began that journey into recovery, I could finally stop blaming the relationships around me and instead start healing them. Today I know I am a good mother and wife. I have gone to any lengths in order to heal, while still allowing my children and husband the space they have needed for their own recoveries. Anyone who comes to Shades quickly realizes there are a number of people running around with the last name McCarty. For years, my husband ran an oil company in west Texas. When I was growing up, my daddy had been an oilman, too. You could say our family business had long been about drilling into the dirt, looking for gold, but what the McCartys used to call oil prospecting, we now call recovery. And we've learned how to do it together.

The Dance of Addiction

The Great Law of the Iroquois states that "In every deliberation, we must consider the impact on the seventh generation." Though this concept is often applied to the environment, I believe it can just as easily speak to the health and well-being of our families. For many of us, we are forever looking backward over our shoulders at the choices and mistakes of our fathers, mothers, and grandparents. In that, we often forget about those who have yet to come, our children, our grandchildren, and the many generations who will inherit the earth, and also our teachings.

Sadly, for those living in denial, we are like actors in a Greek tragedy, each playing out those world philosophies and family dynamics whose lines we know by heart. We demand that everyone around us play their part—for some they are the lead players, always drawing the attention of those around them; for others, they are the duet filled with tearful monologues and parting moments; and then there are the supporting roles inherent in an ensemble cast.

These patterns work to balance out the chaos and instability brought on by the addict, and the rest of the family learns a troubling set of character traits in order to do so. Below you will see that these roles are so typical, they can easily be defined and broken down, as any cast of characters might be. They are archetypes based on the oldest of human instincts, and without fail, the family members of an addict will assume one role or another in order to uphold the family dynamic.

As you read through their descriptions, identify your role and those of your family members (both in your childhood and present family dynamics). Looking back at those letters to your parents, recognize how your mother and/or father supported these roles in your childhood. In reviewing the different characteristics, see which traits you've picked up in order either to maintain your addiction or to alleviate the consequences of someone else's. We would not play these parts if we didn't need to. They are as much about survival as they are about denial, offering the addict, the enabler, and their children ways by which to cope with confusion. Sometimes the roles aren't perfectly played, and often one person might play more than one role. In some cases, you might be the addict; in others the enabler, the scapegoat, or the mascot. I played so many of these roles that at times I didn't know whether I was addicted, enabling, or just trying to escape. Pia Mellody, the great leader in codependency studies, once explained, "In a functional family . . . the adults are able to identify their own needs and wants . . . and they can ask other safe people to help them meet that need or want." For the dysfunctional family, we do not know how to ask for help; we know only how to manipulate. Once I saw how I played all of these roles to get what I wanted or needed, I could begin to change my behavior. And over time, so did the rest of our family.

The Addict. When Patty was brought to Shades of Hope, she was only about nineteen years old, but she looked closer to ninety. Frail from anorexia, covered in a big wool dress in the middle of summer, she could barely move around without the aid of the staff. Her parents had been trying to care for her for years, and though at times she would get closer to a healthy weight, she would inevitably fall back down. By the time Patty came to us, she weighed sixty-four pounds and was addicted to starvation. An addict participates in her addiction because she cannot *not* participate in it. As much as she is intellectually aware of her behaviors, as Patty was once we stabilized her, she is still overcome by the compulsion to engage in the disorder.

Even after we were able to move Patty out of her critical zone, she was still battling to stay around ninety pounds, at which point her mother began to ask when they could take her home. Taking care of an addict gives the whole family its identity, and as much as the family members want that sick person to become healthy, they also find themselves feeling untethered to their roles, lost without the gravitational pull of the addict's need.

Patty is what we call the Identified Patient (IP). The IP is the primary suspect in the dysfunctional family, demanding help and attention from everyone in his or her sphere, crying out either silently or with a resounding tone. Different people in a family can become the IP, but the structure of the family is set up to take care of and to cater to that individual, making the addict the focus, allowing the family to ignore any other issues, even other addictions, that might be occurring in the home.

Who is the addict in your family? Is there more than one? Even if there is one identified patient, are there others who use that IP's addiction to disguise their own? How does the addict continue to maintain his or her dependency? And does he or she also play another role in the family dynamic?

The Enabler. Meet me. Like Patty's mother, as much as I wanted RL to get sober, I also relished the power his addiction gave me, and the freedom it afforded me from looking at my own troubles. Enablers are often the easiest ones to spot. They are tired, acting as though they are responsible for everything and everyone. They can't remember when they last had fun or didn't worry, because their sole focus is protecting the addict from the world while simultaneously begging for the addict to change. They have ulcers, headaches, digestive problems, backaches, high blood pressure, heart problems, and are often nervous and irritable, taking prescription drugs for their depression or anxiety. They think that if only they were better, the addict would quit. They are addicted to the addict.

Often one of the biggest challenges in recovery is the addict's family. Their focus has been on the needs of the IP for so long that when that person becomes healthy, the rest of the family does not know how to respond. In Patty's case, her mother wanted her to come home, get a job, jump right back into normal living, but once we got to know the family dynamic, it became clear that the mother needed her daughter home more than Patty needed to be there. Patty's mother had left her full-time job years before, and since then her life's purpose was to be Patty's nurse.

This is what we call total enmeshment. Patty's mother felt so bad for her, she pitied her little soul; she just wanted to hold her close—nurture her—but she was not letting her find her own two feet, and in the process had begun to ignore all the other relationships in her life. Her husband, her son, and her career were all second fiddle to the caretaking of Patty. When we began to work with the family, it became clear that there were many other issues that they had been able to ignore because of Patty's illness.

That is the thing with addiction: Both the addict and the enabler are so wrapped up in it that they are not available to anyone else. My concern with RL's drinking far outweighed all my other responsibilities. I would stand at the window, waiting to see whether he was coming home, sending the children to bed early just so I could keep my watch, and even when they would get out of bed and tug on my nightdress, wanting their mommy, my focus was entirely on waiting for those car lights to appear, signaling RL's return.

I could not be present to my children because my whole identity was based on whether RL was sober, and in the end, our whole family got sicker than he ever got. Our children were without parents. RL had his booze, and I had RL and food. We were both so focused on our addictions, our children would get left behind. We often disregarded our children's emotions just as we hid from our own. Unable to see and make right where we had hurt them, we both retreated further into our co-dependency and addictions.

Reviewing your own family dynamic, throughout your childhood and today, who has played the enabler? Often we learn to enable from one or both of our parents. Did one of yours fit the role? And do you play it today? Do you perhaps have enablers in your own life? How do they protect you from the consequences of your addiction?

The Family Hero. For a long time, I used to say that we were waiting for my oldest daughter, Karen, to be born just so she could take care of the rest of us. The hero is the caretaker of the family, often considered the "good kid." They are high achievers, they do well in school, they follow the rules, and they seek approval from adults and peers for their achievements.

Heroes are determined that they can "fix" the family—trying to make everyone look good through their accomplishments. They will play Mommy or Daddy to the younger siblings, and often act as a surrogate spouse for the addict or enabler, depending on their gender. In our house, Karen always held a special place in her father's heart. Whereas I beat him with violent words and even the vacuum hose, Karen would lovingly take care of him, showing a patience and kindness that I could not find in my frustration. Because the child is not weighed down with the same responsibilities as the parent, he is able to offer the family more tolerance than the addict or the enabler, and use his abilities to take the focus off the family's disorders. While my other kids were out causing mischief or lost in their own worlds, Karen participated in all the normal fun and functions of childhood and adolescence. She was in 4H, she went to the prom, and she became the evidence I needed to prove that we were just like everyone else.

Sadly for most children raised by addicts, they are forced to play roles beyond their actual age, causing them to mature far too quickly and relinquish their childhood before they ever have the opportunity to experience it. The hero becomes a "little adult," and grows up to perpetuate the same unhealthy cycle, because he was not allowed to properly pass through the development phases of childhood, adolescence, and adulthood.

Who is the hero in your family? Which sibling took on this part? Or did you? How has this hero tried to maintain the outside appearances for your family? And can you see how this role exhausted him or her as he or she bore the weight of someone else's addiction? Do any of your children play this role? What burden do they carry?

The Lost Child. In Patty's family, her brother Charles had been ignored for so long, his needs and development put behind the tragic consequences of Patty's behavior, he ended up finding his own addictions. Charles went to rehab less than a year after Patty came to Shades—his drinking and drug use already significantly dangerous at the age of eighteen. Patty's parents were shocked to find that their other child, the one who had always seemed to fly under the radar, was also battling a life-threatening disease.

Lost children don't talk, trust, or feel. They try to be good, but it's never good enough to make things better. They feel guilty and inadequate because they try so hard to change the family dynamic but are ultimately powerless over it. The lost child is often a daydreamer or a loner. Having little experience to live in the world, they don't receive the support or nurturing they need to help them make friends or socialize. They are prone to allergies, asthma, bed-wetting, and accidents, and find relief in fantasy and their own addictions in order to "escape the family."

When she was growing up, Kristi was the one who got lost in the mix in our family. Though she later took over the role of hero from Karen, she spent her early years adrift in her little world. The rest of our family was so consumed by their own troubles, I'm afraid we didn't do much to invite her in. Karen and Kim would be fighting; my oldest son, Kelly, would be off with friends; RL and I would be dancing with our addictions; and Kristi would be alone in her room, playing by herself.

As Kristi entered her teen years, RL and I began to get into recovery—he with his twelve-step program, and me with Al-Anon. Between our meeting schedule and my addictive behaviors, Kristi was once again abandoned, left to her own devices and feelings of isolation. Recovery is not about neglecting our responsibilities in order to heal, but rather learning to once again take care of our families and ourselves as a whole. Patty's family experienced the same. Once they stopped focusing on Patty and began to focus on the roles they had been playing as a family, they were finally able to begin addressing those deeper core patterns and dysfunctions on which the addictions had thrived.

As you think about your family, who has played the role of the lost child? How have they removed themselves from the family dynamic, becoming invisible amid the drama and confusion of the addictive home? Who was the lost child in your childhood, and is there one in your life today? How can you begin to recognize this family member, inviting him or her back into the fold?

. . .

The Scapegoat. The scapegoat is caught up in the idea that he is not as good as the hero, and since he can't compete, he withdraws and acts out, figuring negative attention is better than no attention. Scapegoats may run away, behave promiscuously, or get into alcohol or drugs. They are often hostile or defiant and feel they have been abandoned or rejected in some way. They have trouble being honest and participating in intimate relationships. They play that negative tape so loud in their heads that they can hear nothing else, seeing everything through the perspective of those messages—their life, their family, and themselves.

When Kim was growing up, I was determined that all the girls wear dresses and look feminine, and she would have none of it. As a child Kim was ornery and stubborn, and once she entered her teen years, RL and I knew that we were going to have some real trouble on our hands. By the time she was in her twenties, Kim was addicted to drugs and alcohol and weighed less than a hundred pounds. We tried for years to help her by putting her in rehabs and hospitals. We always left our door open for her to come home, desperate to manage the costs of her behaviors so she wouldn't have to. But once I went through treatment, I realized what a disservice we were doing Kim, protecting her from her consequences. Instead, we sat her down and explained that she could no longer stay with us unless she was willing to get help, and when she wasn't, we had to say good-bye.

Over the next few years, I lost whatever slim relationship I had with my daughter. We did not speak to each other, and though I cried and prayed about her every night, I came to a place where I had to let go. Even when I knew Kim was living on the streets, as she ended up in psychiatric institutions and suffered from suicide attempts, I knew in my heart that God was holding her. I had surrendered my power. There was nothing I could do but have faith that one day Kim would come home.

That surrender is not easy. The guilt that goes along with raising and watching a child battle addiction is overwhelming. There is no greater pain than to watch your baby suffer. You cannot help but obsess over every decision and action that might have led to your child's illness, drowning yourself in remorse and fear over what you could have done differently.

After a decade away from us, she finally returned. She was a stranger to me at first, but then as we both began to share a program of recovery, we found that the things we had most despised in each other were the traits we both shared. Today Kim is one of our top counselors at Shades, and a daily reminder to me about what can happen when we finally relinquish our control.

Who is your scapegoat? A brother, a sister, a son, a daughter, you? He or she can be the addict, or even take on another role, like lost child, but often their behaviors are nothing but a cry for help, begging for the love and care they are not able to find in the home. Is there a way for you to start changing your behaviors to either stop playing the scapegoat or start nurturing the child or sibling who does?

The Mascot. For every sick family, there is a member who acts almost impervious to the challenges everyone else seems to be facing. This "mascot" brings comic relief to the family, doing anything for a laugh, gaining security and control in order to get attention. She is protected by the family and is often not told the true story. Though mascots feel fear most of the time, they cover it up with laughter, addicted to bringing relief to the family through their humor and easygoing attitude.

My son, Kelly, has always seemed immune to the dramas in our family. He is outgoing, successful, a pleasure to be around, but he is also always performing. Kelly seemed to grow up in the light, immune to the illnesses and addictions we all hid behind, determined to be different.

Like most mascots, he did his best not to affirm the family's addictions, living in a deep and entrenched denial about who we were, believing instead in the family we could have been.

Mascots can make everyone believe that they are happy, that everything is fine. They are experts at the masquerade, and their outgoing personalities can convince anyone that they are managing their lives on the surface. But they still suffer the same effects as everyone else in the addictive household, and are often masking their own addictions.

Growing up, was there a mascot in your home? The class clown, the hyperactive brother or sister, or were you the one who was always able to keep the plates spinning, entertaining others so they couldn't see the pain inside? See who played this role and ask yourself if he or she is still playing it. How does this charade serve him or her?

For many of the folks who have come through Shades, their families demonstrated varying degrees of addiction and abandonment, entrenching those old philosophies in emotional silence. They promised themselves they would never end up like their parents, trying to take a different course, yet still ending up in the same place. Instead of the drink, they picked up cake. Instead of sex addiction, they found themselves restricting their food. Instead of abusing their children, they released the anger and rage through purging.

Once you begin to honestly look at your family dynamic, recognizing those patterns that have played out not only in your relationships, but also on your plate, you will begin to model new behaviors for everyone around you. You will be able to relinquish your old role within the family dynamic. You will be breaking the shackles of the old paradigm, transforming the life you lead today and helping to transform the generations yet to come.

FOUR

Body Image

The group sat waiting for Perry to speak. It was four days into the six-day intensive program, and we had just finished up a body-image exercise in which Perry had been asked to draw what he thought his body looked like. Hanging up on the wall was a large piece of butcher paper with the illustration, a strange block-shaped image over which another client had traced Perry's real shape on the same sheet of paper. Perry's body looked like that of a normal man—though perhaps in need of losing seventy to ninety pounds—a far cry from the shapeless form he had originally drawn. I gave him a few more moments to respond, knowing silence is hard on everyone, reminding them of the thoughts they cannot voice, and the fear that runs through this work.

Perry also felt the pressure, and finally broke out of the shame he was stewing in. "I don't know why I see myself that way; I just do. I look in the mirror and I don't even feel human. I've never really felt human. I just feel like some strange blob moving through the world."

Perry had suffered a number of suicide attempts before finding his way to Shades, which was evident in the portrait he had drawn: absolutely disconnected from his own body, from humanity, and from life.

According to the Bible's story of Genesis, God "created man in his own image; in the image of God He created him; male and female He created them."

From the get-go, it was our human form that set us apart from the other animals, defining us as man and woman, and requiring us to use the earth's natural resources for our survival. And yet we turn against this gift in disgust, hating our bodies, refusing to see them as marvelous systems of movement and life, instead perceiving ourselves as lifeless forms made of fat, cellulite, imperfect skin, and empty weight.

We focus on the extra flesh on our thighs, the thick skin of our arms, a butt that we no longer recognize as our own, and we despise ourselves all the more. Many people are either obsessed by that reflection in the mirror or they can barely look at it. But both experiences are born out of the same sense of self-obsession—this idea that our value is based in the image we see in the mirror, and not on the contents it contains.

In *The House on Mango Street,* Sandra Cisneros's book about coming of age in Chicago, the main character, Esperanza, tells her friends that Eskimos have thirty different names for snow. One of her little pals replies, "There ain't thirty different kinds of snow. . . . There are two kinds. The clean kind and the dirty kind, clean and dirty. Only two." But another little girl, Nenny, disagrees. "There are a million zillion kinds. . . . No two exactly alike."

Growing up, I was absolutely convinced that there were only two body types: clean/dirty, skinny/fat, pretty/ugly, good or bad. I was so convinced that I was dirty, ugly, and bad, it didn't matter how much I hated being fat; that was my type, and it was my prison. For years, I lived in that small, dark box of my body image. Every once in a while someone would come by and rattle the cage, hinting that there might be another way, and a little bit of self-love would creep in. But I had become an old woman in that body, unable to accept any other kind of life. Until finally I just couldn't live in that lonely box anymore and I came out, and when I did, I discovered that there weren't just two body types in this world; there were billions, and each one was absolutely different and deserving of love.

The Mirrored Plate

Once Perry began to open up, we saw how his body image had been created not to mirror the divine, but rather to cover up his pain. Perry had grown up in a lonely household, forced to take care of his sick mother since he was eight. When he should have been out playing with friends, engaging with others, Perry lived in isolation, turning to food for friendship. It was his best friend, more reliable than anyone else, including his mother, who had fibromyalgia and was dying of a rare autoimmune disease. After going to the school nurse one afternoon, he realized that he had gained fifty pounds in one summer.

He later explained, "I was afraid of everyone—boys and girls— especially when I got into high school. I wasn't able to talk. It felt like I was stuck in the recesses of my mind, and as much as I wanted to reach out, I just couldn't; I couldn't make myself engage. I started staying in more and more and would just sit in my room obsessing over food. The food was everything."

Our body is our temple, given to us by God so that we may be of use to our fellows. It was not designed to be beaten with food, tortured with purging, left to atrophy without exercise or proper nutrition. It was created to participate in harvest and fellowship with others, so that we may procreate and continue on this earth. Yet when we turn to food for company, we hinder our ability to engage with other humans.

Perry later told me, "There was nothing in my life that didn't revolve around what I ate. If someone invited me to a movie, it would depend on whether I was restricting or bingeing that I would go. Because I couldn't be around food if I wasn't allowed to eat it, and that often meant I couldn't be around people."

Every choice we make around food relates to the other choices we make in our lives. In order to identify that connection, however, you first must have some clarity about your relationship to food today. Have you ever participated in any of the following behaviors, even just once? Allow yourself to see the choices you are making for your body, the patterns you are repeating on your plate.

- Do you typically eat breakfast? Lunch? Dinner?
- Do you snack? Often? At what time of day or night?
- Do you ever hide or sneak food?
- Are you having difficulty sleeping?
- Are you getting up in the middle of the night to eat?
- Have you ever eaten out of a trash can?
- Do you binge? How often?
- What kinds of food do you binge on?
- Do you purge? How often?
- Do you abuse laxatives? How often? How many times a day?
- Do you have any side effects from your laxative abuse?
- Do you abuse diuretics? How often? How many times a day?
- Do you have any side effects from your diuretic abuse?
- Do you exercise? How often?
- Do you restrict your food—eating less than your nutritional needs in an attempt to lose weight? How often? How much?
- Has your relationship with food damaged any of your relationships?
- Have you ever had to face any negative consequences due to your eating habits?

Just as we cannot see the truth in our hearts until we are willing to hold up the emotional mirror, so, too, we cannot see the real truths about our body until we take a fearlessly honest look at our plates: what we are eating, how we are eating, and why we are eating.

As we continued to work with Perry, he told us, "For so long, the food was the only thing I had control over in my life. My mother died, and even when I started working and got married, I felt so powerless in my life. But the food was mine. I owned it, I controlled it, and I knew what the results would be from eating it, even if I didn't like them."

If you have been living under this illusion of control, believing that you are in charge of your diet when really it is the diet that rules you, there is only one way to stop manipulating your plate. You must create a healthy meal plan, one not based on calories or fat grams, but rather on the nutrients you need for sustenance. This is not another diet, where we believe we either work the system perfectly—never straying from its rules—or we cheat one little bit and decide the whole thing is off. We *will* err, and when we do, abstinence is about changing that recording in our heads so we can tell ourselves, "It's okay. I made a mistake. I am going back to my plan right now." Healthy eating isn't about rules; it is about changing your lifestyle, your belief system, so that you can always begin again.

Looking back at all of your answers, I ask you not to beat yourself up, but to see without judgment those parts of yourself as objective facts, not subjective feelings. They are the building blocks of recovery, and as you look over them, I want you to start thinking about how you have used food to cope with your feelings:

- When have you eaten, binged, restricted, or purged because of how you were feeling in that moment?
- How have you used food to respond to the following emotions: anger, fear, pain, loneliness, shame, guilt, and joy?

- How has the food only made you feel worse?
- How has it made you angry, fearful, in pain, lonely, shameful, guilty, or happy?
- What does food do for you?
- What does it do to you?

Reaching Your Quota

Years ago, I remember hearing RL tell someone that he didn't drink anymore because he had reached his quota. The same goes for the food addict. When people start the program at Shades, the complaints about the food are unending: It's too bland, it's too spicy, there are too many vegetables, there aren't enough vegetables, the portions are too big, the portions are too small, and, at the end of the day, it all comes down to the fact that we just have too much choice in our lives.

Sarah was an attractive advertising executive from Boston with short red hair, striking blue eyes, and an extra forty pounds she hated like the devil. And she thought she could teach us all a thing or two. By her third week, Sarah had written us a long, professional letter describing the changes she would like to see in the food offered at Shades of Hope: more variety, a midafternoon snack, some chocolate, and more food before bed. Our team couldn't stop laughing when we read the letter, seeing how the addict's mind thinks itself so powerful that it can manipulate the people it asked for help. I can only imagine what would happen if we started adding Cap'n Crunch before bedtime, and chocolate-chip cookies for an afternoon snack.

I approached Sarah and asked her about the letter. She smiled demurely, shrugging. "I just thought you should know what we all would like."

"Mmmm . . . is this your diet at home?" I asked.

"Sometimes."

"And how did that work for you?"

Sarah stopped.

"Sarah, we take away your control with food so you can see just how little control you have. I know you want to live healthier; otherwise you wouldn't be here, right?"

She nodded.

"So why would we offer you the same food that rules your life at home? I'm going to guess you've had enough chocolate and bedtime cereal to last you a lifetime."

Sarah glared at me.

"Sarah, what's really the problem here?"

She smiled sadly. "I'm hungry."

Hunger is the number one complaint of most of our clients. But the meal plan offered at Shades actually meets all nutritional requirements. Physical hunger comes when we don't have enough calories or nutrients in our system to survive. It's our body's way of telling us we need to be fed. But for so many food addicts, hunger is about seeking the same relief the alcoholic finds in the bottle, the gambler at the casino. The meal plan we offer at Shades is used to create new habits, not rooted in the pleasure and relief we have always found in food, but in the nutrients and calories we need to subsist.

The question for you is: Have you reached your quota? Haven't you eaten enough unhealthy foods and gone on enough sugar binges to last the rest of your life? Because most food addicts have had the fine meals and fast-food fixes, eating in excess at times, at others starving themselves through whatever pop diet was on TV. It is time to surrender the idea that you can continue to eat however you like and still assert control. The food has dictated your life for long enough; now is the time to reclaim it.

Viewing the Body

There are countless body types in this world, and each one of them is beautiful in its own right, each serving a unique purpose on this earth. Unfortunately for many of us, we think love is based on the size of our thighs, value is weighed on a scale, and our intrinsic worth comes down to the dressing room mirror at our local mall.

My whole life I believed that once I lost the weight, my identity would change. Becoming someone else, I thought everything would be better, different; I was going to lose twenty pounds and be a better child. I was going to lose fifty pounds and be a better mother. Lose one hundred and be a better wife. And there were times when I would lose the weight. Getting on a drastic diet, I would restrict for a short period of time, and the pounds would come off. And then they would come right back on.

Weight and value were so inextricably linked, my whole identity was centered in the size of my dress. I was either fat Tennie or skinny Tennie, but either way, there was always the lurking notion that I was still a fraud—a big girl hiding out in another woman's body. My closet was like a department store, because I had the same clothes in sizes zero to fifty-two. Weight loss would become a project, and it would feel wonderful for the first part of the time, buying new clothes even though I knew it wasn't going to last. When I was thinner, people would tell me how great I looked and ask how I did it. But then six months would go by, I would gain it all back, and I'd be embarrassed when I would run into the same people, seeing their surprise that I had gotten so heavy again.

But no matter how much weight I lost, I could never think of myself as thin. As I began to work with others, I realized this had very little to do with size, and everything to do with perspective.

Carla sits on the floor silently weeping. She is a news anchor who lives in San Diego. With thick brown hair and a flawless complexion, she exudes confidence to all who meet her. She is staring at her piece of butcher paper, the tears streaming down her face. As she looks at the image she just drew and the one traced from her body, her real form takes up only a third of the space of her illustration. Despite her multiple degrees, blooming career, and a very beautiful figure, Carla had just drawn the body of an obese person.

"Carla?" I interrupt her crying. "Do you want to tell us how you feel?"

The tears only come harder as she explains. "I just. . . I look around at all these people in my world, and they're so thin, and I feel like a monster next to them. I try so hard to be a size two, not even a size zero, and it seems like I can't get there. I don't want to starve myself, but how can I not? I feel so fat and gross."

She looked up at that paper again, and I could see in her eyes the same self-hatred and disappointment that I had carried when I was aiming for a size twenty-two. For many food addicts, our body distortion is so off that we don't know what we look like. In order to begin to live in the objective reality that recovery requires, and not the subjective lies on which addiction feeds, you must begin to get back in touch with your body, seeing what your real size is. I want you to look at the following body diagram, the figure's shoulders, arms, legs, waist, and then imagine your own body. Then draw what you think you look like against the figure (see page 92).

Where do you think your body is larger? Where are you smaller? Are you taller than the image, or shorter? Where do you see similarities between you and the figure? Where do you see differences?

Don't look at yourself in the mirror. Simply close your eyes and draw the size you feel your body is. If you want to keep your eyes closed as you draw, feel free. There is no right way or wrong way to do this. This is about recognizing how you view yourself in your own mind, rather than the image reflected in the mirror.

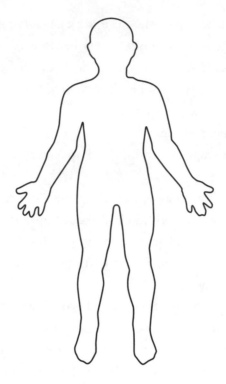

You can also perform at home the exercise we do at Shades. Get a large piece of butcher paper, lay it on the floor, and, based on the idea in your head, try to draw an outline of your own body. Once you are finished, ask someone to help you. Lie down on the drawing and ask your friend to outline your exact actual silhouette. Then stand back and look at the difference between the two shapes.

Look at the image you have just drawn, and see if you can view it with the compassion and tenderness you would offer a small child. Be kind with the image and with yourself for drawing it. Ask yourself whether the drawing looks right. Is it realistic? Often we will see people draw images that don't even resemble human beings, but rather cartoon figures of what a person might look like. They draw themselves twice as large or twice as small. Grown women create images of themselves that look like adolescent boys, and anorexic men view themselves in large, monsterlike proportions, all unable to bring their self-love to the table.

Before Carla left treatment she told me, "I finally realized that it's not about the number; it never has been. It's about whether I am willing to love that person in the mirror."

Everything we think or do comes from our imagination. If we put garbage in, we get garbage out, so we must reprogram what we are putting in, in terms of both food and ideas. We must be willing to look in that mirror and begin to see ourselves from a new perspective, as terrifying as that process might be. When I was living in my addiction, my self-loathing got so bad it was hard for me to comb my hair in the morning or put on lotion, let alone see myself in the mirror; that reflection was a stranger, an intruder in my life. I treated it as a form to be neglected and abused, not cared for as the body with which I had been entrusted, the temple for my soul.

Holding Up the Mirror

For so long, we have let our plates be our mirrors, basing all our opinions and ideas on who we are on how much is on our plate. We disconnect from our bodies by overconnecting with food, allowing it to be our primary relationship, paramount to all others. In order to heal, we must become present to the relationship with self, taking the focus off the plate and facing that person in the mirror.

One of the exercises we did with Carla, and one I will now suggest for you, is to get yourself a large paper bag, like a grocery store bag or something that would be large enough to fit over your head. (Make sure it is paper—no plastics or other materials.) Then cut out two holes for your eyes and a slit for your nose so that you can breathe easily. Find a room in your house that has the most mirrors and privacy; most likely this will be your bathroom. Take about fifteen minutes—preferably when no one else is home—and go in there and lock the door, making yourself feel as secure as possible.

Once you are alone, undress yourself. I strongly suggest getting entirely naked: no socks, no underwear, no jewelry. I want you to push yourself, but not to the point where it's unmanageable. Try to get as unclothed as possible while still remaining comfortable. Next, take that paper bag and put it over your head and look at yourself in the mirror. Here is your chance to engage in absolute self-love, leaving behind any of those negative messages and thoughts that block us from connecting with ourselves. Instead, focus on what your body offers you, bringing in compassion and avoiding judgment.

Begin to recognize how this miraculous system of movement—your legs and arms and torso—define you as a human being, setting you apart from all the other animals on our earth.

What are your first reactions?

Do you see what your food addiction has done to you? And can you look past that and begin to appreciate the body with which you were blessed?

Start with your shoulders. Are they sloped? Are they strong?

What does your skin look like: taut or relaxed with time?

Can you feel the weight of your purse, your briefcase, the grocery and shopping bags that are so often digging into your shoulders? Can you thank your shoulders for all the hard work they do for you—lifting boxes, groceries, children? Do you feel like you are carrying an invisible load, that the weight of the world is upon you? Thank them for that, too, for carrying both the physical and emotional weight of life.

Then move down to your chest. If you are a man, look at your pecs. Are they pulled tight or do they hang loose? Did they help you in sports as a child? Do you use them in physical activities today? Lifting weights?

Playing softball? Do they help you to raise your children into the sky? Do you feel your heart beating in there, guiding you through life? What does it have to say? For women, take a moment to feel your breasts, thanking them. If you are a mother who has breast-fed, appreciate them for providing food and have gratitude for their health. Love them for being yours. If you have had or have breast cancer, say a little prayer that they may stay healthy or continue to heal.

Now take a look at your stomach. Remember, you are not here to criticize. Having done that your whole life, you are here only to love. Put your hands on your belly and flex your muscles, seeing how your stomach helps you to move. Thank it for helping you to eat, for carrying your food and emotions. If you are a mother, thank your belly, and everything it contains, for also carrying your children. Relaxing, hold the soft, round part that all humans and most animals carry. Your stomach is not supposed to be hard; it is supposed to be supple. Look at it in the mirror and say, "Thank you, belly, for being mine."

Moving down to your hips and thighs, stop for a moment and think how blessed you are to have been born with hips. These joints between your pelvis and femur are responsible for all human movement, from sitting to standing to walking to running. Watch your hips as you lift your legs, seeing how they move. If you are a woman, imagine how life passes through them. Look at your legs, touching them; pay attention to their movements. What do your thighs feel like? Your calves? How have your legs served you? How can you appreciate them more? Thank them for their strength, for helping you to walk upright, for giving you the freedom of movement we so often take for granted.

Reaching your arms up into the air, look at your biceps. Feel free to flex and have some fun with your body; move your arms around. Dance. Laugh. It is a rare day when we allow ourselves to be so free. Think of all the things your arms have lifted—from small things like a pen, to luggage, to children. Wrap them around yourself and remember all the times they have been wrapped around another. Holding yourself for a moment, experience what true self-love feels like, recognizing the comfort you have sought in food but have always held within. Thank your arms for all they have done for you. And then, before you are finished, look at your hands and feet—how precise they are, how complete. Make a promise to love your body with the kindness and generosity you would offer a child, seeing in it the child you once were, and the man or woman you have become.

Before you get dressed, stay just one more moment. If you have started to cry throughout this process, let yourself cry. If you have started to laugh, laugh. This moment is just for you. You can feel whatever you want, but remember this is not about building or playing that negative tape. When Michelangelo sculpted his masterpiece, *David,* he began with a big block of marble and had to find the divine form of David within. I ask that you now do the same with yourself. Get rid of all that marble of negativity and all the voices that tell you, "You're fat," "No one can love you," "You've already blown it, so just keep eating." Chip all of that away and see yourself as the divine form you are. Be grateful for your shoulders, your chest, your stomach, your hips, your thighs, your arms, your feet, and your hands. They were created just for you, and all they ask for is your attention and care.

When you are ready, take off the paper bag and look at yourself in the mirror, into your pupil, the dark area of your eye, and say, "I love you." If it feels strange, try again. Say it until you can feel it. Repeat this exercise every couple of days or weeks. Self-love is a powerful force, an eternal gift, and it will flow in all directions once you allow it.

PART THREE

Decision

Dear Lord, be good to me. The sea is so wide and my boat is so small.

—IRISH FISHERMAN'S PRAYER

⟲⟳

FIVE

Spiritual Problem Defined

I was blessed to have embarked upon the journey of recovery with a number of distinguished mentors beside me—one of the most important being Joe McQuany, a pioneer in the twelve-step movement. Up until his death in 2007, Joe spent over half a century teaching others how to recover from alcoholism and substance abuse, driven by the belief that "we are born for one purpose . . . to help one another." After his passing, I became great friends with his personal assistant, Billy, who had worked for Joe for many years. Not long ago, Billy was staying at our house, and as he, RL, and I had dinner, he remembered a night when he had been dining with his former boss and dear friend. They were at a recovery convention, and in the midst of their meal, guests at the conference kept coming up, trying to speak with Joe.

Billy told me, "It became ridiculous. We couldn't put a bite in our mouths because there was someone else standing there, wanting to shake Joe's hand. We had been traveling all day, and I had gotten in my head that we would be able to settle down to a nice dinner before Joe had to speak. I had planned it all out; I was Joe's assistant, after all, scheduling it as his rest period, not more time on the job. I started to get really irritated, and eventually stood up to leave, deciding I would go to my room and eat there until Joe spoke, but Joe stopped me, explaining that this was part of our work. We had to always make ourselves available, even when it was inconvenient. He joked that we would rest when we died, but until then we needed to stay where God had sent us."

Billy laughed, remembering his reaction as he sat back down and asked Joe, "How do you always accept life on life's terms? Don't you ever get annoyed by people?"

Billy told us that he wasn't sure whether Joe's response was referring to Billy's own frustrations, the folks who were barraging them, or both, but he replied in his deep Southern accent, "Billy, there is no reason to waste our time and energy over things or people we can't control. All we can do is live in acceptance, finding gratitude. We are fortunate to carry this message, to finally be joyous, happy, and free. God has always wanted as much for us. We're supposed to be free human beings."

Sadly, for most of us, we have never allowed ourselves to be free. We have been imprisoned our whole lives by those ancient belief systems, and addicted to anything that would take us out of the present—our present circumstances, our present feelings, the present disappointment that our plans aren't going accordingly. The food serves as judge, jury, and warden, as we protest that we can handle it, we can lose the weight anytime, we are in control.

The Big C

Rachel brooded in the large circle of the weekly group therapy meeting we hold at Shades. She has been living in a size-eighteen dress since she was fourteen years old, but swore this had been by her choice; it had always been her choice.

"I'm the one who puts the food in my mouth," she declared. "I'm the one who pays the price. I'm in charge of the food, I decide how much I weigh and how much I eat, and if I really wanted to, I know I could live differently."

I allowed someone else in the group to respond, knowing that there were enough clients present who had once held the same idea, and had seen the fraudulence in it. One of our younger clients raised her hand. Grace is a beautiful young woman with delicate features and a spritely attitude, who, at the age of twenty-two, was mature beyond her years. After a terrible experience with bulimia and overeating, she ended up at Shades and, having already gone through the program, was then attending college, a great testament to recovery.

She looked at Rachel with compassion. "I used to have the Big C, too. It's called control. I was as addicted to it as I was to the food, thinking the only thing I could manage in my life was my eating disorder. I knew I couldn't control my family, I couldn't control what happened in the world or at school, but I knew that I could control what I ate and what I did with my food afterward. And then one day, I didn't want to be doing that anymore. I didn't want to be bingeing to the point where it hurt. I didn't want to see that sick woman in the mirror, and yet still I couldn't stop. That's when I realized I didn't control anything, least of all my food. It absolutely controlled me."

We want what we want when we want it. If we could control our relationship to food then we would lose the weight with ease, always able to decline the second helping, sticking to the fitness plan, staying with the diet. But as much as we strive for a healthy life, as much as we try to control what goes into our mouths, we find ourselves back to the same old habits, doing what we always did, and expecting something different.

Ultimately, control is the biggest lie we tell ourselves. We believe that we are able to direct our lives like a captain commands his ship, yet we fail to recognize the power of the ocean. I can walk outside today with the best-laid plans, get in my car, and punch a destination into the GPS, but I cannot prevent the teenager from joyriding through a stoplight, just as I cannot control the traffic on the highway, nor the brewing storm. What I can do is structure my life in such a way that I am organized for all those outcomes: having insurance for the accident, patience for the traffic, and awareness of the weather.

Before I was abstinent in my eating disorder, I was like Rachel, convinced that I was in control of everything. I wanted desperately to be loved, successful, honest, and kind, and yet I found myself acting in ways that only sabotaged those efforts. It was as though the more I tried to control life, the more I was thwarted by it. In my frustration, I believed that food was the only thing over which I had jurisdiction. I decided what I ate, determining how much I would gain or lose, lording it over the only thing in my life I felt was predictable.

I had been determined that my way was the right way, even when it was making me miserable. There are no words more humbling or difficult to utter than "I was wrong." I see clients come in every day just wanting to be "right," but if they were right, they wouldn't be in treatment. They wouldn't be overweight or underweight, struggling for balance. For me, the road to recovery was paved with admitting that I didn't know everything, that I could get lost just as quickly as the next person, and that I needed help. I finally conceded that there was no way I could do this alone, and eventually I began to appreciate the freedom that powerlessness brings.

Alpha and Omega

Each of us has walked a personal journey with the concept of God. For some, they grew up in a religious household, either embracing or rejecting the traditions of their family; for others, God was a distant fairy tale, exposed by the cruel realities of life as a con as big as Santa Claus. But either way, whether through religion, agnosticism, or atheism, we have had a spiritual experience. Even not believing is believing. Though we might speak here of God with ease, for many folks the term is laden with opinions, fears, a queasy feeling that they are being fed something they don't wish to swallow. Before we go any further, I am going to ask you to try to let go of your preconceived notions about what God is or is not. Begin to see this concept not necessarily as the God of your childhood or local church (although both are more than fine), but rather as a higher power of your *own* understanding.

For us food addicts, we have long been ruled by a higher power without giving it the thought or credit it deserved. We have made food our god—turning to it in good times and bad, and asking for its love and omnipresence no matter how many times we might turn away from it in an effort to lose weight, to eat healthier. We have prayed at its temples of grocery stores, restaurants, fast-food chains, and the corner market, but now you have the opportunity to give up the god of food. It is not your alpha and omega: your beginning and your end. You can find a new higher power, a guiding, creative intelligence that forms the foundation of our existence. If you allow it, it can be a great well of strength from which you may drink, finding wisdom and faith where before there was only food.

We use the term *God* for lack of a better word (and throughout this book, also the pronoun "He"), but in that we understand that God does not need to be anything more than you are willing to make Him,

Her, or It. To quote the great philosopher Herbert Spencer, "There is a principle which is a bar against all information, which is proof against all arguments and which cannot fail to keep a man in everlasting ignorance—that principle is contempt prior to investigation."

So I ask you to set aside any contempt, allowing yourself a new experience in faith, with no judgment, no intolerance, just the belief that God comes in many forms: your best friend, a lightbulb, the sky, birds, and the great natural beauty of our Earth. If you are willing to see where God might be revealed, you will find that He is everywhere and in everything, just waiting for us to finally surrender control.

Snoopy Faith

When I entered Al-Anon, the twelve-step program for families of alcoholics, I was exhausted by decades of unsuccessful attempts to get RL sober. Tired of playing God, I realized it was time for me to get a new one. I needed to find a God concept that didn't speak to the self-will that ruled my thinking, but rather to the spirit of love I had seen through the folks I met in Al-Anon, and through the kindness I had received from them. I was out walking one day after I returned home from a meeting; the sun was just beginning to sink down in the big Texas sky, and I started to skip. As an overweight child, I had never skipped, but there I was, like a lunatic, skipping down the street. I felt like Snoopy, like a carefree pup, just moving through the world, and I decided in that moment that that was who my new God was going to be: Snoopy.

For the first time, I saw my higher power not as a concept handed to me by others, but as an energy that I could either tap into or ignore. I loved Snoopy's energy—his innocence, his optimism—and I knew that was what God meant to me. I stopped seeing spirituality and religion in the same context, and I began to understand that God could have many faces. It seemed silly, but it also seemed like the kind of endearing love I needed from my God at that time. I needed a God who not only spoke to my adult side, but also to the child who had never been able to trust in anything or anyone.

At first, my faith grew slowly. I was taking tentative steps toward relying on someone else besides myself. My sponsor in Al-Anon instructed me to pray every night and meditate every morning. At first, I resisted. As much as I had gone to church, I didn't really know what it meant to stand alone with my higher power and me. But then I began to see that if I woke up every morning and wrote out my prayers, and did some reading in a meditation book, my day would go much better.

And since I joined that program in October 1968, I have woken up to a morning meditation almost every day. Sometimes my vision of God has been quite clear, and other times I just think of that old Snoopy dog, some easy illustration of what I believe God to be: kind, loving, loyal, and honest. And much like the Charles Shultz character, my Snoopy God has also grown. In the original comic strip, Snoopy had no owner, no voice or thoughts. He lived in a doghouse in search of someone to take care of him. But as the comic developed, Snoopy grew to obtain an owner, find his voice, and discover that the view was much better from the roof. And so my God started out as a fictional cartoon dog, but over the years, that Snoopy faith has grown into a sustaining presence, teaching me that God can be found both in the church and on its roof.

Spiritual Anxiety

Every time a food addict picks up a candy bar or a Big Gulp, she is thumbing her nose at the spiritual world, proclaiming her reliance on food over faith. Every time someone stays in an unhealthy relationship, she is eschewing the love of God, convinced that it will not be enough to sustain her without the relationship at hand. Every time we go to the mall and walk out spending more on our credit card than we know is responsible, we are turning our back on faith, believing that we will be sustained only by material goods rather than spiritual fulfillment.

I have a dear friend, Pat, who often tells the story of Adam and Eve with her own interpretation. She explains that when God's first children entered the Garden of Eden, eating from the Tree of Knowledge, it was not the apple nor God that descended shame upon them; it was Adam and Eve. They were the ones who quickly covered up, embarrassed by their own humanity. They believed that they had done wrong and cowered from God and His impending judgment. God was simply confused by their behavior, asking why they were hiding, reassuring them of His love. But Adam and Eve were so convinced of their wrongdoing, they confessed to evil before they were even condemned. And we are no different.

When I first met Jolene, she was everything I had wanted to be when I was a younger woman: thin, attractive, with thick, long hair and a perfect French manicure. On her third day in, she knocked on the front door of my house and asked if we could talk. I knew that she was supposed to be at dinner, that our staff was probably looking for her, but Buffalo Gap is about the size of a modern-day Wal-Mart, so I knew it wouldn't be hard for them to track her down.

Jolene came into my living room, sitting down on my couch, her legs crossed neatly; she declined my offer of tea or water. I sat down in a chair next to her, waiting for what was about to come next.

She began, "I don't belong here."

Bingo. This is normally everyone's sentiment.

"Uh-huh," I replied.

"I feel like I made a mistake. I thought I had a problem, but really it's not that bad; I just didn't want to be rude, and I thought I should let you know."

I explained to her that she could check out whenever she wanted, but that she would need to speak with Cam, our executive director and my daughter-in-law. I smiled. "But that's not why you're here."

"No, I wanted to be polite; you seem like a really nice woman, and—"

"Most people think I'm a bitch by day three," I interrupted. "Tell me something: Have you ever felt like you belonged?"

Jolene stopped. I could hear her breath escape for a moment as she tried to plaster that smile back on.

"Stop smiling, Jolene. Just answer the question. Where do you belong? With your face in a toilet, staring into your own mess? You think that's what God wants for you? That's His big plan: Jolene gets to vomit up her food every day; she gets to shudder with her own violence, her own self-hatred?" I could feel her beginning to tremble as I reached across and put my hand on hers. "What kind of God would want His children to live in a bathroom?"

And that was when the tears began. Jolene told me how none of this felt right to her, that it felt strange and raw, as if her skin were being peeled off. She just wanted the comfort of home, but really she was aching for the purging, not knowing how to live outside of her world of shame and self-hatred.

She had spent her whole life trying to get good—going to church, reading the Bible—but she saw her disorder with food as a sin, not a disease, assuming God would punish her for her behaviors. She didn't even think she could ask for His help. I understood. For a long time I felt trapped in the same dark hole of doubt, believing that miracles were for other people, for the addict next door, but not for me. Addiction flourishes in this alienation—telling us that others can get better, but that we are different, unique, and special. We believe that recovery won't work for us, or we're not sick enough to need it. It whispers into the ear of the addict, "Even if there is a God who could help, wouldn't He have done so already?"

It never enters into our eating disorder that God can remove that mental obsession with food if we are willing to ask for His help, and not assume His judgment. We pray to God while fearing Him like the devil, denying His existence while simultaneously disbelieving His love for us.

I asked Jolene whether she might be willing to have a new experience in God, to see Him not as a judge, but as a protector, as a source of light and strength, guiding her along her destiny, asking only for her cooperation along the path.

She meekly said, "I don't know that a God like that would have me."

"You belong here, Jolene. As uncomfortable as love is, why don't you let us love you a bit longer until it doesn't hurt anymore? And I bet if you start asking God for help, and become willing to receive it, you'll see how much God loves you, too. You might even be able to realize that it isn't God who's been doing the judging."

She smiled and nodded. "It's me."

It's me; it's you; it has always been us, never God. Our higher power only loves, as much as we don't know how to be or sit in that. We go chasing the food in order to receive consolation, fearing that we will never find comfort elsewhere. But when we begin to recover, as Jolene went on to do, we find there are no mistakes in God's world, only lessons to become more able human beings, to love one another with more presence, and to finally learn to love ourselves as God did on the birth of our creation.

SPIRITUAL ABUSE

I sat in the annex building where we conduct the six-day intensive program; the little room in which this powerful work is conducted suddenly seemed way too small for the folks sitting in it. They are not morbidly obese; in fact, most of them are close enough to their healthy weights, but they are all women who have struggled with using food to remove them from life's challenges. And they are all psychotherapists. On the first mention of the word *God*, four hands shoot up. I'm not even sure whom to choose first. I nod to a woman who sits cross-legged. With her casual appearance in sweats, her hair in a ponytail, she belies her age and stature, as Marta is the director of psychology at a major university. She tells me, "In my experience, I have seen as much damage done by religious people as I have seen them do right. I don't know that bringing up God to treat eating disorders really speaks to the sociopsychological nature of addiction, and more than that, it is sure to bring up all kinds of issues surrounding spiritual abuse and religious dogma, from which vulnerable people should be spared."

The rest of the room nods. "Yes, yes, what she said." And, surprising them, I nod my head, too, because I have treated enough survivors of spiritual abuse to understand that having a new God concept can be incredibly difficult when your previous idea was warped by those you thought were there to protect you.

Spiritual abuse can take place in a number of different ways. Sometimes children don't even need to leave the house to experience it. Spiritual abuse can happen when parents become like a god for the child, or when a child is preached one thing but then sees the parents living something quite different. The child thinks that his parents are immortal, that everything they say is the word, and then, when he doesn't see that exhibited in his parents' behavior, he loses faith in God.

Spiritual abuse in the church takes a similar form. I have worked for years with ministers, priests, and chaplains who are exemplary members of the faith community, carrying the word of God with humble arms and kind mouths. But when church leaders abuse their power, they act as gods for their believers until they reveal themselves as flawed humans, causing the believer to no longer trust.

I have seen hideous abuses of power in almost every faith, but I have also seen great salvation. I learned early to recognize where religious people were right, to take what I needed from their prayers, their rituals, and then to incorporate them where I saw fit. For many people, church has always been home, and it still is home. For others, they have much work to do in order to forgive the religion of their childhood, and to find that they are now free to believe in what they wish: either their previous faith, or a whole new experience of the meaning and understanding of God.

As Marta feared, this abuse can be a great obstacle, and one I frequently come up against, but it is not an impossible one. Our relationship with a higher power is always there, always open to renegotiation and reinterpretation.

God Is Love

Many centuries ago there lived a Catholic priest in France who tired of preaching that anyone who died outside the Catholic Church would be barred from heaven. One day, he was blessed with a mystical revelation wherein the spirit reminded him that God is love. The spirit forever changed him, and the priest began to minister to all who lived in his village—not just to the Roman Catholics, but to every faith and lifestyle, knowing that if God is truly love, then there could be no rejection.

The Buddha furthers this idea, describing "health [as] the greatest gift, contentment the greatest wealth, faithfulness the best relationship." Unfortunately, most food addicts spend their time in relationship with food, not faith, and certainly not with others. That doesn't mean that we don't show up for our loved ones in all sorts of ways: blindly paying bills, making shopping lists, showing up for the company Christmas party, our daughter's middle school dance. We once again get by doing the basics of our responsibilities, but are we really present?

Our spirituality is the breath of all our relationships. It is in the bond between two people that the spirit of God most clearly shines through. The love of a mother toward her child, the friendship between two women, a man's love for his wife—these are all spiritual experiences. Every time we love someone, we are doing God's work. And every time we fail to show up for those relationships, and for ourselves, we fall out of step with the spirit of the universe.

I remember one afternoon many years ago when I was helping Kristi with her homework; she was only eight at the time. As we sat at our decorated dining room table covered in matching place mats, napkins, salt-and pepper shakers, ceramic bowls and bottles to hold every condiment under the sun, I could hear her talking, telling me a story about her day. She sat there chatting away, as eight-year-olds do, with their wonderful gap-toothed smiles, sharing all their new life experiences: friends and boys and schoolyard pranks. Suddenly, she stopped talking; looking at me curiously, she asked, "Mommy, do you ever listen to people?"

It was a heartbreaking moment, because I didn't listen; I didn't know how. While she had been sharing her little world with me, I was staring at the ketchup bottle sitting on the kitchen table. It was not in the porcelain dish I demanded my children put it in, but had been left in its original plastic bottle. As Kristi continued talking, I had gone through rage at the children for leaving the bottle out, to intense hunger, thinking of all things I could put the ketchup on. In the space of five minutes, I had gone from considering abandoning my family for daring to leave out a ketchup bottle, to figuring out how I could go binge-eat while Kristi was alone at home, to worrying about one of the place mats on the table, which hung a half inch off the side, as though daring me with its insubordinate behavior.

In that moment, not listening to my sweet, freckle-faced girl who needed her mommy to pay attention, I was incapable of being present to anything but my own obsessions. God is not in yesterday; nor is He in tomorrow. He is not in the place mat nor the ketchup bottle nor the terrifying idea that we can get up and leave anytime we want—God is now. And He is found in the love we share with others.

Spiritual bankruptcy occurs when folks can no longer participate in those relationships. After a while, that lack of presence not only takes us out of the relationship, but it sends us fleeing into shame. Like Adam and Eve in the garden, we are so disappointed by our own behaviors, we live in fear of those we love most, unable to connect to them in the deep and present ways that true love and faith demand.

We all have a path to spirituality, no matter how different our roads might look. Once we can see that God is personal, that God is for everyone, we can begin to build a relationship not based on the ideas of others, but one that feels right and befitting for us. As you look at the following questions, see how your behaviors are blocking that path. How has your relationship with food not only interrupted your relationship with God, but with others elsewhere in your life?

- How does practicing or not practicing your relationship to food hamper your spiritual relationships with other people and with God?
- How is your spirit burdened by your behavior?
- What does your relationship with God look like today?
- Can you feel the presence of love in your life?
- Can you feel the presence of God?
- How do you feel when you are practicing healthy eating behaviors? Do you feel that you are better able to participate in your relationships? With others? With God? With yourself?

Make a Decision

We are not idiots. We wouldn't eat, binge, or starve if it didn't work for us. For a long time, those higher powers of food, control, lookism, and codependency served us like the most rigorous of spiritual practices. But since that first failed diet, the first weight-loss video thrown to the back of the closet, we have lived in a place where that initial salvation has increasingly waned. The skinny phases become just as painful as the fat ones, always reminding us that our successes, our health, our quest for and attainment of perfection are tenuous, if not altogether futile. And we're really, really tired. Tired to the point that we are willing to take action.

I remember when I came to that crossroads, recognizing that either I continued praying to chili dogs and ice-cream cones, or started believing in a God that would fill that hole in my soul with a much greater breath. I made room for God to come in and do His work; I began to see miracle after miracle, understanding that God often appears in the form of someone else, someone who helps me to do something I cannot do on my own. Once I began to trust in those relationships, I was able to trust in God.

On the last day of the six-day intensive program, we take the clients out to a local restaurant, giving them their first chance to order and eat from a sizable menu offering everything from healthy meals to tempting choices. We come almost every week, so the waitstaff knows our meal plan well enough to act as coaches for our clients, helping them pick and choose from their menu, making new choices they have never made before: ordering soup and salad, requesting that half their meal be put in a to-go container before they are even served, making sure the chicken is baked and not fried. The ninety minutes we spend in that restaurant can be as spiritually transformative for clients as any Sunday morning they have spent in church. They are getting to see the first fruits of their labors, feeling the freedom to make the right choice, even if they are also free to make the wrong one—and we have certainly seen our fair share of folks who immediately place an order for a cheeseburger, onion rings, a large piece of cake.

Recently I sat with a new group of clients who, after being in our six-day intensive program, removed from their phones, computers, and families, were now surrounded by food and people, taking the first wary step into their new lives. One of those clients, Liz, sat next to me, perusing her menu, laboring over each choice. I could feel her fear, smell her self-doubt as her eyes scanned the desserts, all while her conscience whispered, *Salad*.

I leaned over. "The chicken quesadilla here is one of the best in Texas. We always get the half order."

She looked up at me as though I had just written her a million-dollar check. "I can have that?"

"You can have whatever you want, Liz. You just need to ask yourself why you want it."

She looked down at the menu as though it were a sacred scripture. "Because I'm scared. I don't know how to do this; I feel like if I make the wrong decision, I'll be doomed. It will all be over."

"What will be over?"

"My life." She shivered. Liz had been yo-yoing for years, from 178 to 328 pounds, and though we had recommended she stay longer, she was adamant that she needed to be home, explaining that her husband, her children, her job all needed her. Six days was all she could give.

"It might be over," I offered. "Although it's not going to be the molten chocolate cake or the full order of quesadillas that's going to do it. But believing that you're doomed will."

Liz closed the menu; breathing in, she looked at me. "If I stay, then everyone will know that I'm sick; they'll know that I'm not . . ."

"Perfect?"

For the majority of her stay, Liz had been committed to the idea that she did not have an eating disorder, that she was just trying to lose some weight, and hoping that Shades of Hope could help her with that.

"Liz, perfection doesn't come through our controlling everything; it comes through our having faith that God has a path for us, and it's our decision whether we want to take it. Do you think God brought you to this earth to have a panic attack every time you look at a menu, or does He want you to be free from that exhausting obsession going on in your head? Because I can hear it in there, Liz. I'm getting worn out by it; I can only imagine how you feel."

Liz smiled wearily. "Exhausted." Tired of hiding behind her responsibilities while never being present for them, sick of being controlled by menus, of waking up every morning wondering whether there was something more, of spreading the mustard on her daughter's sandwich like a zombie, in that moment, Liz had made her decision. She knew that home and God and love and family would never satisfy her until she could let go of that feeling that she was doomed, and begin to find a new freedom without the counterfeit safety of food. She decided to stay for the six-week residential program, and began to try on a different life for size.

SIX

Finding a Spiritual Solution

When I was eight, I found God—or rather, I found His congregation. I remember sitting outside my house, the terra-cotta dust that draped across west Texas bustling across our yard. I scratched my leg and looked at the small hairs beginning to sprout out of it—all while the voices inside my house got shriller and shriller. My mother and father fought like cats in heat, howling so loud the whole neighborhood could hear. I couldn't stand to be inside, yet I was terrified to leave. I had it in my head that sooner or later one of them was going to try to kill the other, and if I wasn't there to stop it, who would? So I would keep watch outside, waiting for my father to threaten my mama, and thinking about all the ways in which I would try to protect her. But on that day I just couldn't listen anymore. I sat there as long as I could, and then I stood up. I was almost 150 pounds, so it wasn't easy for me to get anywhere in a hurry, but I started walking just as fast as I could, trying desperately to put space between me and the rage that lived within our house. After a couple of blocks, I realized I didn't even know where I was going. I had no friends, no money, no means of transportation. I knew I wasn't running away, but I also felt as if there were somewhere I was supposed to be, as if there were a place out there that would help and protect me, if only I could find it.

Since you can't very well throw a rock in our parts without hitting a Baptist or a Pentecostal church, it didn't take me long to stumble into the latter, entranced by the hymns that were echoing down the road. I knelt in a pew, on the hardwood kneeler, praying that someone or something would come and remove me from my childhood, take me out of the screaming, the sound of broken plates, and the ever-present fear of violence. I began to hear the minister speak; reading from the Bible, he quoted Psalm 23:

> The Lord is my shepherd, I lack nothing.
>
> He makes me lie down in green pastures, He leads me beside quiet waters,
>
> He refreshes my soul. He guides me along the right paths for His name's sake.
>
> Even though I walk through the valley of the shadow of death, I will fear no evil,
>
> for You are with me; Your rod and Your staff, they comfort me.

I knew right then what I hungered for: I wanted that spirit of the Lord. I wanted to lie down in green pastures, beside quiet waters, and fear no evil. I waited until the end of the sermon, when they offered that anyone who wanted to find salvation could come to the front and be baptized. I walked up, absolutely terrified, but hoping that somehow these folks might be the comfort I was seeking. As they dunked my head under the water, an old woman clutching me to her breast, all I could think about was whether my mother set aside dinner for me back home. It was the beginning of a lifelong battle between the spiritual life and one consumed by food and fear.

When I walked back through our front door that afternoon, I proclaimed to my mama, who was through fighting and had returned to drinking on the couch, "I've been saved!"

My mama looked at me with her cool, drunk eyes, a sly grin on her face, and asked, "Saved from what?"

I wanted to shout out, "From you, from Daddy, from this horrible, miserable life!" but I was too scared. The wind had been quickly removed from my sails, and I went into the kitchen, relieved to see a plate cooling on the stove, baptizing me in a way that church never could.

Though I would go back to church for decades, trying new religions, pushing my children into all the classes and ministries I could find, I always felt like I did that day, after rushing home to my mother's dismissal: that the light of God did not shine upon me no matter how hard I demanded Its presence. By the time I made it to treatment, I had twisted my concept of God into a knot so tight it was better fit for a noose. I went back to the idea that I was one of two types of snow: the skinny, good, clean kind, or the fat, bad, and dirty. I believed I was in God's grace as long as I was sticking to my diet, staying within my budget, being a good wife and mother, and I was outside God's grace every time I yelled at my daughters, ate their school lunches, or argued with my husband.

It took my going to treatment to realize how self-centered that idea was, that I alone was so special, so important in the eyes of God that he would thrust me from His love because of a pack of Ho Hos. How we define God is a direct reflection of what we think about ourselves. When my God was a cruel and judging phenomenon that damned me over my eating habits, that was because I was cruel and judging, damning myself at every turn. My God did not echo the stories of the Bible, the Torah, the Buddha, or any other religious teaching, but rather my own negative tape.

Coming Home

Everyone's experience with faith is different. My daughter Kim walked into treatment with no God at all, not even wanting a God. But then she realized that she believed in many things of this world without knowing how they worked—electricity, radio waves, love—so perhaps finding God wasn't actually about finding God; it was about seeking Him. Since her own early days in recovery, she has built a powerful relationship with her spirit world, reminiscent more of the Native American tribes that once lived in Buffalo Gap than the churches in which she was raised. Through that, she began to see that God was not necessarily an external being, separate from man, but rather a spirit who could always be found within.

A few years back, Kim went to a sweat lodge with a Native American shaman she had begun working with to help underprivileged teens. When she came home, she told me that as she sat in the dark, hot lodge, watching her thoughts emerge and disappear like dreams, the shaman had leaned over and whispered to her, "Grandfather's got you. You're safe now. You can come home."

When we finally return to that innocent and loving faith (for me it was Snoopy; for Kim it was nature), when we begin to recognize that quiet light within ourselves, our understanding of God is revolutionized. Kim told me later that it was in that moment in the lodge that God revealed Himself to her; He was in her grandfather, her ancestors. Whereas my faith has led me back to my church, her God led her back to her childhood faith—where she saw God in her family, in the lace of the trees, and in the wondrous beauty of nature. She felt like she had been returned full circle, and just as the shaman said, she was home.

For someone who came in believing that God was dead, Kim has found God to be very much alive in her life, present in the work she does at Shades and in her own recovery process, but that took time. More often than not, the spiritual part doesn't come right away. First we must give up the substance or process; we must experience the pain of abstinence—only then is there room for God in a food addict's soul. Instead of praying and relying on the higher power called food, folks are able to turn their will and their lives over to the care of God. By stepping just a little bit deeper into faith, we are able to ask for God's help in removing the obsession with food. God can and will if He is sought, if only we are able to rely on His love, and not on the habits we need to break.

New God Concept

Anne Lamott once described a film in which a group of old Gypsy women danced, flaunting the abandon of age. "[They had] time for all those long deep breaths, time to watch more closely, time to learn and enjoy what I've always been afraid of—the sag and the invisibility, the ease of understanding that life is not about doing."

God has offered us this freedom since the day we were born, handing us quite literally the sun, the moon, the earth for our appreciation. And he gives us bodies with which to dance under those stars and moon, and upon this earth. Sadly, we are all so busy doing, so busy worrying, so busy dieting, crying, complaining, judging, criticizing, weighing, eating, purging, starving, dying, that we watch life go by and don't really let ourselves live it until we are craggy old Gypsies with nothing left to lose.

The moment I met Steve, I could tell he had probably laughed only a dozen times in his whole life. He had once been a compulsive overeater, getting up to five hundred pounds, and then, after receiving the Lap-Band, swinging the other way to anorexia/bulimia. When he finally made it to Shades, he was down to eating one cup of soup a day, or he would binge and purge, keeping nothing down at all. Steve had grown up in a very conservative church, and though he was still part of his faith community, he felt as though he didn't belong.

Though Steve was a successful lawyer, though he had close friends and mentors around him, there was one thing he just couldn't come to terms with: the sexual abuse he suffered as a child. He had struggled with it for years. Though he had wanted to be in an intimate relationship with someone, he didn't know how to because of it. He lived in so much shame because, as a child, he had heard in church that the acts that took place were wrong, and he had carried that with him his whole life. Though intellectually he knew the abuse wasn't his fault, in his heart he considered himself a sinner.

While he was at Shades, he wrote to a minister who had worked at his alma mater, asking him his thoughts on God, and how one could have a new experience in religion, no matter his past. The minister, Burt Burleson, wrote back, and this is what he said:

For now . . . know that you are a unique and unrepeatable expression of the divine. God's essence is within you. This is what is most true about us all. The deepest levels of self are united with God. This is our authentic self that, while covered up, is undamaged and kept in God's grace. Remember we can surrender and receive what is. "This is my life . . . this is the world, . . ." Simply be present to this. . . . All we need is here. God is present here and now in this reality. *You are loved.*

When you live half a block from a treatment center, you are used to getting calls late into the night, but more often than not they are because someone is threatening to leave or to harm himself or herself. The late-night calls are very rarely good news. But that night, when my phone rang at nine thirty p.m., I knew the tears on the other end of the line were from joy.

Steve told me, "I thought I was damaged, Tennie. I thought anyone who knew of God would say that I was, that I wasn't supposed to be here, that I shouldn't have been born, but that's not what this letter says. It says that I've been in God's grace this whole time. He's been holding that poor little boy in the palm of His hand, hasn't He?"

I started crying myself, and the next day, when Steve handed me the letter, it was as though he were holding the Word of God, faith beaming from his eyes so strong he would have made a believer out of anyone who saw him. Steve finally had been given permission to exist—that letter offering him a vision of God that was protective and present, caring for mankind despite the pains and trials we might suffer.

And now I give that same permission to you. Whatever your concept of a higher power might be, here is your opportunity to describe it. It's a rare day when we really get to look at what God means to us. Even while we sit in a church pew, do we truly understand what that experience encompasses, what our relationship with our higher power reflects? Do you see how God should mirror that authentic self, and not all the judgment and pain covering it up? If your current higher power is the one you wish to keep, please do so. No need changing partners if the one you have works. If you feel you need a new God, here is your chance to explore what you are looking for, what sort of spiritual traits and ideals you would like for your new vision to embody. This is all up to you.

After you answer the following questions, feel free to draw or write a poem, to go out and take some pictures of the world outside that reflect your understanding of God. Allow this to be a creative endeavor.

There is no right or wrong here, and you may create whatever portrait you wish.

- What does my higher power look like?
- How does He/She speak to me?
- When have I seen God's work in my life?
- What would I like my higher power to do for me?
- How do I want God to reveal Him-/Herself in my life?
- What aspects of faith/love/trust/acceptance would I want that higher power to exhibit?
- What does having a higher power mean to me?
- Do I believe that this power will take care of me?

God Is Not a Codependent

Marisa was one of our clients at Shades of Hope when we first opened our doors in the late 1980s. After she left, we continued to talk on the phone. At first I acted like a sponsor for her, but over the years, we have both come to help each other. I have leaned on her to help me with my abstinence from overeating just as much as she has leaned on me. Whereas I have had the grace to be surrounded by folks in recovery, Marisa lives a long distance from any twelve-step meetings, and has had trouble staying connected with other recovering food addicts. She runs a large agricultural company in Kentucky, overseeing more than a thousand employees. Doing global business in a well-trodden man's world, Marisa has been caught between her crazy work schedule and the buffet tables that come with business life, fighting to stay abstinent from her own compulsive overeating.

Last year she called me in hysterics, crying so hard I thought her cat had died. Finally she caught her breath. "I feel like I just can't get a break. I try so hard; you know I do. I'm praying and meditating like a fool, and still I break my diet."

"What are you doing on a diet?" I asked. Marisa has been on a healthy meal plan for many years, eating solid, regular meals, well aware of the difference between dieting and recovery. As we both know, a diet has a goal, a number, and a time frame; recovery is one day at a time, with an eye on forever.

"I just wanted to lose the weight. Tennie, if it's all about God, then why isn't He helping me?"

I've asked that same question before, expecting God to show up just because I hit my knees and asked Him. And not that prayer isn't a powerful act, but it's hard to be in action if you're only on your knees. "Marisa, I'm sure God is trying to help as best He can, but what have you been doing to help? Did you ever call that young lady you met who was struggling with bingeing?"

Marisa broke from her tears to defend herself. "I've been busy."

"Well, sweetheart, God doesn't drive a parked car. You've got to at least put it in neutral. Try to take some kind of action other than another diet. How can your God reach out to you if you can't reach out to another?"

Marisa exhaled on the other end of the line. "I called you."

"I know, but how about you go call that other girl? And instead of asking for help, try to offer it."

They say that you can't have esteem unless you perform esteemed acts—sharing the light of recovery and offering to someone else the gift of healing that was so freely given to you. For a long time, I wanted to bitch and moan to God and anyone who would listen, thinking that all my troubles would be removed if I cried hard enough about them. But God is not a codependent; He is a gentleman. He can't help us if we aren't willing to get up off our knees and do the next right action, recommitting to our meal plan and finding a way to be of service to others and ourselves. Marisa made the right choice that day. She called someone (me), and because of that, she ended up calling someone else: that young lady who was feeling just as depressed and disappointed in herself as Marisa.

Prayer and Meditation

There are a million ways to meditate, and everyone must find the path that fits them the best. For me, I have found that writing down my hopes and prayers helps me to set my intentions for the day. Sometimes I might do my morning meditation for fifteen minutes; other times I might take an hour, but I believe that if you give yourself at least that fifteen minutes every morning to connect with a higher power of your understanding, you will be transformed. Whether you take that time to read from meditation books, to practice breathing exercises, or to tap into a religious or spiritual practice that fits your concept of God, play with ideas for how you can spend this time. Try it for six weeks, and by the end you will be hard-pressed not to see where God shows up in your life.

At night, take a moment to say thank-you for your day. To think over all the things for which you are grateful. If you want to write them down, put them in your journal. Once you have started the meal plan, you can also use this time to look at where you have strayed and where you have stayed on course. Our evening prayers can be used for evaluation as much as meditation. Offer yourself a few minutes to breathe in deep and think of all the right choices you made that day, and then if you made some mistakes, think or write down how you could have done them differently. If you need to apologize or rectify the situation, write down how you should do that. By taking this nightly inventory, we can better understand and put in perspective the day we just experienced. And then we can turn it over to God, ask for His forgiveness and help, and offer our gratitude for another abstinent day.

Letting Go and Letting God

Nothing gets removed from me without claw marks. Even after I experienced the power and light of a loving faith, my first instinct was not to turn over my life's concerns to the care of God, but rather to control every aspect of their development. Though God has proved to me time and time again that He doesn't intend to drop me on my ass, I still try to assert my role as captain of the ship, believing that without my guidance God will be lost. Faith takes practice, and over time I have seen that if I am willing to be guided by God, as opposed to demanding which way the ship turns, my course runs much more smoothly, and with much less trouble.

Many years ago, when I decided to create an eating-disorder clinic, I found myself torn between opening it at the Serenity House or striking out on my own. My instincts whispered to me that there needed to be a place where people with eating disorders could be treated independent of other addicts, but I was so afraid, terrified that I would be making a professional and financial mistake to leave the safety of Serenity.

The board of directors got tired of my hemming and hawing, demanding that I sign a contract to run the clinic out of their treatment center. They wanted me to commit myself to their program, staving off my own treatment center idea for years, if not for good. I was sitting in the middle of the board meeting, listening to the directors explain to me the freedom I would have, the support, and yet something in me said it wasn't right. They slid the contract across the table, and just as I was preparing to sign, my assistant came in the room to tell me my daughter Karen had called. She was in labor.

I told the directors that I would sign upon my return, but first I had to get to Lubbock for the birth of my first granddaughter. Leaving Abilene, I couldn't believe the timing of that moment. As much as I knew that I would be well compensated for staying, I just wasn't ready to sign.

I arrived at the hospital in time to see the delivery of Karen's first-born, my first grandchild, a beautiful baby girl with emerald eyes and pink skin, just another reminder of God's grace. Afterward I walked around the hospital, taking some time to think. Passing a room filled with people, I could tell a twelve-step meeting was in progress. I stepped inside, surprised to find it was actually an Overeaters Anonymous meeting. I sat down with tears in my eyes, overwhelmed by the precision of life when we move in the direction God guides us.

"God will show us what we need," the speaker said. "He never directs us where He wants us to go until we are willing to give up where we are at."

Once again, God shone a light on my path, removing the obstacles. I knew the choice I wanted to make: It wasn't about being secure; it was about being of service. I knew in my heart that people with eating disorders deserved a clinic of their own, a safe and special place where they could confront a disease many did not even know existed. I envisioned Shades of Hope long before we opened its doors, knowing it was time to go where God was directing, believing He would support and protect me along the way.

Liz, the young mother who had a near breakdown at our local restaurant, ended up staying at Shades of Hope, participating in our six-week residential program. After a couple of weeks, it became clear that she was trapped so deeply in that negative tape, believing that God echoed its judgments, that she was deaf to any other perspectives being offered.

One afternoon I took her outside. It was a hot Texas spring afternoon, summer threatening from a close distance. I turned her toward the sun, asking her to close her eyes. Though defiant, she did it, squinting tightly, her body wound up like a coil.

"Liz, relax. You are standing in the sunlight of the spirit. That warmth on your face, the slight breeze on your skin, the sound of the crickets chirping, that is your connection to God. That is God. He is holding you so tight, no matter how alone you might feel. He is always there, shining down on you."

I could see the tears slip down from under her closed eyes. She stood there for another moment as I joined her, remembering one of my favorite scriptures in the Bible—a mantra I have used for years: "Be still and know that I am God." When I meditate, I break it down: Be still and know. Be still. Be. Before recovery, I did not know how to be still in my own skin, let alone to be still and know that God is working everything out just as quickly as He can.

Finally Liz looked over to me. "We're free, aren't we, Tennie?"

I nodded. "We are. We were always meant to be."

༼ ☉ ☉ ༽

SEVEN

Recognizing the
Divine Self

*A*ccording to Alice Miller, author of *The Drama of the Gifted Child* and a researcher on childhood development, "For the majority of sensitive people, the true self remains deeply and thoroughly hidden. But how can you love something you do not know, something that has never been loved? A little reflection soon shows how inconceivable it is to really love others (not merely to need them), if one cannot love oneself as one really is. And how could a person do that if, from the very beginning, he has had no chance to experience true feelings and to know himself?"

For so many food addicts, they have grown up with this erroneous notion that they are wrong or have less value than their peers. They create this vision of themselves not grounded in the roots of their reality but rather in the falsities of their perception. For some, they believe the lies told to them by others. For others, they believe the lies they tell themselves. But for all, they ignore one supreme fact: They are a divine and perfect child of God. All of us were brought here for a purpose. Some people are here to better the world, to be of service to the whole of mankind. And some of us are given much more specific missions—assigned the heavy task of parent, of daughter, of one among the many.

But in our addictions, we lose sight of that divine purpose. We lose ourselves to the food, and forget about the tasks at hand. We ignore the relationships. We forgo our dreams, believing that we are not capable or not good enough to be present to our own lives.

For those of us who suffered abuse as children, we fight another battle with our post-traumatic stress. We lose ourselves to the abuse. Buying into the shame that was put upon us, we consider ourselves damaged goods, denying the miracle that is our lives. And we end up blaming everyone for this loss. We become victims and, quite unwittingly, repeat the cycle of victimization by continuing with abusive relationships and behaviors.

We continue to give away the power that defines that authentic, divine being—because that woman inside who dreams of a healthier life is a very powerful person, and that man who knows he deserves more than a Chinese buffet on a Friday night holds all the keys to a recovered life. But the addiction stops us from seeing that the solution is within. It tells us to blame our mother or our father. It says we can't be right because of our past. It taunts us with the memory of love withheld and pain endured. And we silence that powerful self once again with the buffet, the shopping trip, and the unsaid truths in our relationships.

We must let that past go in order to move into our future. This is not about blaming anyone anymore. Most sick people were raised by sick people who themselves were brought up by sick people. In order to finally release that imprisoned divine self, we have to begin to see that only we can be responsible for the present. We cannot change anyone else, but we can change ourselves. We are our problem. But we are also our solution. Because that divine higher power lives within all of us. And though we may be fallible (all humans are), we are also filled with spirit. There is a great, powerful light that was set aglow at your birth, and which is now flickering within you. Stop for a moment and put your palm to your heart. Connect with that deep sensational energy, that bright light of your soul. Unfortunately, most of us have spent our lives covering that light up. We create this persona of who we think we should be (the happy homemaker, the successful professional, the bed-bound invalid), and we fail to see what we are capable of being.

We use our food as a shield to ameliorate the pain that living in this false self creates. And we ignore the innocent, joyful, spirited self within. All you have to do is watch a child play to see who that forgotten self is—devoid of malice, anxiety, self-doubt, children reach out to strangers with love and curiosity, living in amazement at each new interaction. I know that at the age of four I was as sweet and innocent as any other child, adoring my parents, attentive to my surroundings, filled with questions and laughter and a wide-eyed bemusement about life . . . until my mother had the affair.

When I was growing up, my father was often working in the oil fields, cheating with other women, and returning home to alternately romance and fight with my mother. Mama loved when he came home, but in his absence, and fueled by her drinking, she often found herself entertaining other partners. One of those men was a local neighbor named Mr. Thompson.

The first day Mr. Thompson took my mother and me out on the town, my whole life changed: The sky seemed brighter, the trees greener, amplified by the heightened tension that I could feel from the front seat of Mr. Thompson's car. Mr. Thompson knew you had to pet the calf to get the cow, so that very first day, he took me to a candy store and helped me pick out what I wanted: toffees, peppermints, chocolate bars, bubblegum sticks, jawbreakers. I was overwhelmed by the choice as my mother's lover filled a bag that would never feel so full again. I sat in the back of the car as my mother and Mr. Thompson canoodled, simultaneously falling in love with the candy melting in my mouth. It took me away from the betrayal I might not have known I was participating in, but certainly felt.

In addition to the bags of candy, Mr. Thompson would also offer me compliments, a far rarer and more precious thing. He would tell me I was as pretty as my mama, that all the boys were going to adore me one day. I began to feel like I was having an affair, cheating on my daddy with a much more loving man. Over the next year, my mother and Mr. Thompson's affair continued in motel rooms across our community while I ate candy in the next room, starting a cycle of fear, shame, guilt, and food that I would continue for the next fifty years.

One day, when my father came home, he took me out for a drive, which should have raised a flag for my mother had she been sober enough to pay attention (my father never took me anywhere on his own). Just as Mr. Thompson had, he gave me a bag of candy, driving me around, asking questions about Mama and her friend. With each bite of the candy, the syrup of the sweets coalescing in the back of my throat, and my stomach cramping out of fear, I answered his questions, telling him what I had seen. He calmly drove us home. Later, he said what a good girl I was, giving me the approval he had rarely shown. Though I felt bad about divulging Mama's and my secret, I was as happy as a lark that my father had finally offered me a kind word.

Not long after, my father called Mr. Thompson over to the house. I was sent outside. I was so sick, believing it was my fault; I hid in the bushes, waiting to see what was going to happen next. I could hear the yelling, voices so loud I thought the police would quickly be on their way. My mama's was the loudest, screaming, "No," over and over again, until Mr. Thompson stumbled out the front door, blood squirting from his neck like one of those chickens in Mama Johnson's coop. My father was quick on his heels with a knife in hand, threatening to cut more than his throat the next time.

I crouched down lower in the bushes, terrified my daddy might catch me next. I peed myself from the fear and guilt and the trauma of watching a nice man get hurt because of the things I said. And from that moment, I began to employ the candy, which Mr. Thompson and my own father had used to buy my loyalty, to mitigate my emotions in the aftermath.

The innocence of a little girl had been taken by a group of adults who could no more see the consequences of their actions on a child than they could see them for themselves. Mr. Thompson might have had a slit throat, my mother a broken heart, and my father a sick and twisted revenge, but that little girl walked away more injured than all of them put together.

The Divine Child Within

Childhood, like life, is filled with disappointment. We grow up to find that our parents are only human, other children can be cruel, and that the right amount of candy can bring harmony to the soul. We figure that the only way to manage the whole mess is to try to control it, so at least we don't have to be hurt *and* surprised. We try desperately to create schemes and plans to protect ourselves. If only we were in charge, life would run smoothly. And it's no wonder we are disappointed. It's no wonder we turn to food in consolation, the one thing over which we have power, or rather the illusion of it. We think that because we decide our portions, we are food's masters. And then one day, we wake up and realize that food has mutinied and we are wholly under its charge.

Beneath all these unhealthy survival mechanisms built to help us navigate an unpredictable world lies that sweet, darling child who just wants to be told she is lovely, that she is a good girl, that she is deserving of Daddy's and Mommy's attention. This pure, authentic being is the part of us that still dreams of unfulfilled plans and goals. This is the part of us that aches to try a new hobby, to go traveling, to find another job. This is that secret place that cries out and asks to be treated with respect and dignity. Within each of us lies this source of power and identity. It is the child who says, "No!" It is the woman who stands up for herself after years of being abused by an angry husband. It is the man who finally tries sailing after always loving boats.

This divine self is the root of our reality. It is who we always wanted to be, who we always were, but instead we allowed the negative messages or abuse we suffered in childhood to waylay us. We stood on the other side of that deep spiritual light—blocked by negativity, fear, resentments, and, later, our addictions. That guilt and shame of believing that we didn't deserve lives filled with joy and inspiration is what stops us from living lives filled with joy and inspiration. In our attempt to mute the pain, our addictions also squelch the joy.

Before recovery, all my feelings were like a surgery stopped midway. I was exposed to the world, to all the bacteria and disease, yet never given the time nor the space to heal. Instead I just got sicker as that authentic self was buried under a life history I tried to ignore.

We use our childhoods as the biggest of excuses. I kept my stories like a strong hand in Texas Hold 'Em—never showing what I had but believing it was what made me different. I thought the horrors of my past kept me from meeting my potential. I never talked about the incident with Mr. Thompson until decades later. I told myself that it didn't affect me, that everyone had suffering in his or her childhood, discounting all the pain and guilt that I felt was trapped underneath. I ignored that little girl's pain, and my adult self ended up paying the price.

The child mind is one of the most egocentric on earth, understanding every experience, observation, and message through the lens of self. The developmental psychologist Jean Piaget described it best in his three-mountains task. In this experiment, a child would sit in front of a play mountain range with three peaks, her doll on the opposite side, and when asked which peak the doll was able to see, the child would describe the mountain from her own point of view. Unfortunately, many addicts are trapped in this egocentric stage of development, harboring those old messages like fugitives until the pain forces them out into the light.

Once I began to work through those pains, something in me began to grow up. Though I was already a mother who had raised children of her own, there was still the damaged child in me who had started that negative tape of fear and guilt and pain, and who had never been loved enough to let it go. And though I tried to love my children in a whole and present way, I realized that I could not be present to them until I could be present to myself. I couldn't reach the potential of my career, my family, myself until I started listening to that divine voice within that told me that all my dreams could come true. And that I deserved every one of them.

Sabotage of the Inner Child

By Darryl's fourth day he was ready to leave. I walked up to our main administrative building for our weekly staff meeting and saw him sitting there with his bag packed, looking like a kid running away from home. Darryl was in his early thirties at the time, quite successful in the tech industry, and had been an overeater since he was seven, a bulimic since thirteen. After a failed suicide attempt, his parents pressured him into coming to Shades of Hope, but Darryl was not pleased; ignoring any opportunities to engage with other clients and staff, he spent most of his time sitting in the sun on the same porch where he now sat waiting to go home.

I stopped before heading into the building. "Hi, Darryl."

He replied hello without even looking in my direction, preparing himself for a lecture.

"Where are you going?"

"Home."

"Your parents are coming to get you?" I asked, knowing full well that his parents probably hadn't heard about this yet.

He glared at me. "I'm thirty-three. I'm taking a taxi."

I nodded. "Okay, then. Well, know we're always here for you."

I walked inside, heading to the staff meeting, figuring that, like any angry child, that wasn't going to be enough for Darryl. Two minutes later, Darryl appeared in the doorway of our meeting, the room of counselors looking up in surprise at him standing there, and he standing there just as surprised to find a room of counselors.

"Perfect timing, Darryl." I pulled out a chair for him. "We were hoping you'd join us."

But Darryl didn't move, focusing in on me. "You know, I wouldn't be leaving if you didn't treat me like a child."

"I'm sorry; how are we doing that?"

"Telling me what to eat, what to do, where I can go. I'm an adult; I make a lot of money, you know? You might want to treat your clients with a little more respect."

I nodded, listening to his concerns, and, seeing that he was pleased with himself, I stopped him before he went back outside. "Have you ever been in the hospital, Darryl?"

He looked around the room, knowing that we had all seen his file, that we were aware of his multiple visits to mental wards and intensive-care units.

"Yes." He sniffed.

"And do they let you eat whatever you want, do whatever you want, go where you want to go?" He stared at me as I asked again, "Do they?"

"No."

"This isn't a resort, Darryl. We are here to save your life. Perhaps if you didn't let that little boy inside tell you that you were at a hotel, and listened instead to the adult who knew he was in a hospital, you wouldn't be so mad at us. Maybe you could see that we are here to offer you medical service, treatment for your illness, not rules or lectures or spankings."

That hurt and forgotten child within holds so many addicts back, forcing them to react in strange ways to life. They get upset for no reason, looking to an outside substance or process to rebel, to state their case, to make their presence known. This inner child holds the key to those core issues, and, once the addict begins to look in the mirror, she sees the ways in which that wounded self begs for attention. She is willing to do anything, including sabotage her present life, in order to be heard and healed. The "child" within makes us do these things because she was, and still is, unhappy. Her needs were not met, and she still responds to the world today with the same self-defeating behavior that was inflicted by her parents or the world around her. It is the "child" who:

- Makes us late for work or appointments
- Misplaces and loses things
- Can't get or hold a good job
- Can't reach out and make friends
- Makes us feel that other people are better than we are
- Cannot think of anything to say, or fears we will say the wrong thing
- Leaves things to the last minute so we are always pressured
- Gets sleepy or feels bored so we don't pay attention when we should

- Says, "Don't try; you'll never make it"
- Keeps our surroundings messy and untidy
- Always does favors at the cost of our time and energy so people will like us
- Misreads and misinterprets or overlooks important instructions
- Argues and gives excessive excuses when presented with alternatives or good advice
- Won't let us do what we know is good for us
- Plays the negative tape in our heads
- Marries the wrong person or mishandles our children
- Shackles us to a habit that keeps us enslaved
- Eats too much or smokes too much or drinks too much

Beneath all of these lies lives that authentic, divine self that is being held in God's grace. But in order to find that self, we must first be willing to uncover, discover, and discard everything that is covering it up. We must recognize those core issues and unpack the feelings around them. From there, we can create a new self-concept based not in the deep, dark well of our family histories and negative messaging, but in the true self just waiting to be revealed.

Uncovering the Child

By the time Darryl's Family Week came around, he was ready and willing to meet with his parents, letting them in on the road he took to bulimia, and the messages that fed his overeating. He was nervous to do the family sculpt, wherein he and other clients would act out the dynamic in which he was raised, playing the different roles of father, mother, and sibling to illustrate the messages he heard at home. But Darryl told me that he knew it was time to meet that little boy inside.

Darryl's mother sat in the small annex room where we held the family meetings. She was the first one there, knitting a scarf when I came in. She looked up at me. "I thought Darryl might need a scarf for the cold winters here. I'm hoping to finish this before we leave."

I didn't have the heart to tell her that it wouldn't be getting that cold in Buffalo Gap, but I understood the sentiment. She still wanted to take care of him, reassure him that he would be okay for his stay at Shades. I sat down and, while she knitted, asked her what she thought of Darryl having to be in treatment. She didn't miss a stitch as she replied, "It's weird. The whole thing. He's a boy; he shouldn't be throwing up his food, and even the overeating. We raised him with such healthy things—no sugary cereals, no fast food. I don't understand how he got such a bad habit."

I waited to respond as the rest of the family began to walk in, his father and brother, and then Darryl. Our other therapists, families, and clients in the Family Week program also joined, preparing to do Darryl's family sculpt. We talked for a bit about how everyone was feeling, what was about to happen, all while Darryl's mother continued to knit, speaking only when spoken to. Her needles clacked away until finally I stopped her, asking that she put away the knitting for the sculpt. I watched her back straighten as she complied.

Darryl and three other clients got up and acted out his childhood, telling the story of how, when he was in second grade, his father had received a large inheritance, forever changing their lives. Before he had shared a room with his older brother, and his family devoted lots of time at home to one another. But then they got a much larger house, wherein Darryl's parents lived in one wing and Darryl and his brother lived in two other separate areas. His mother spent her time shopping and decorating. His father was able to invest much more money in his business, taking him away from the family. And Darryl's older brother, who was then an early teen, was off with friends or in his room, now far away from Darryl.

Overnight, Darryl's whole life felt uprooted. He became lost in that big house, alienated from his family and forgotten next to all the accessories offered by their new life. Darryl's parents had not meant to harm him, but his sensitive mind told him he was unloved and unlovable, and he began to eat to make up for it. As there were no sweets allowed in the house (Darryl's mother *was* strict in that regard), Darryl began to binge in secret, creating a disturbing trend that would last into his adulthood.

When we got into the family sculpt, it didn't take long for the inner child to reveal himself. He expressed the messages he thought his family had given him over that period, reflecting their indifference: "You're not important"; "We've got better things to do"; "I'm too busy for you right now"; "You don't deserve to be a part of this family." Now, was that what Darryl's family was saying? Absolutely not, but that was what he was hearing.

Darryl did not see the circumstances of his family from their viewpoint, but rather through the egocentric perspective of a child unable to separate his thoughts, ideas, and concepts from his family's and, similarly, unable to separate theirs from his own.

This work is not about assigning blame. As Darryl began to see throughout his Family Week, his parents didn't wake up and say, "We're going to screw up our child's life today." But through their own inattentiveness to the changes in their lives, they thought that Darryl was as happy as they were about the new home and lifestyle. They were unaware of the pain he was going through, and the pain he carried long after he left the family home. By the end of the sculpt, Darryl found himself curled up into a ball, that inner child more present than he had been in decades. He cried about his loneliness, about his sense that he had been rejected, but in that, he was also able to see how his childlike perspective had influenced those ideas.

This work is not about going back and having a happy childhood; it's too late for that. But you can evaluate that childhood and, through the process, identify the messages that covered up that divine, authentic self within. As you begin to explore what those messages mean, and how they have stopped you from experiencing and fulfilling your emotional journey, you will be able to honor the inner child, growing yourself up into a healthy and whole adulthood.

Using the directional figure below again, think of and write down five to seven adjectives that describe a baby: i.e., *innocent, loving, needy, beautiful,* and so on. Write them all on the figure in one colored pen.

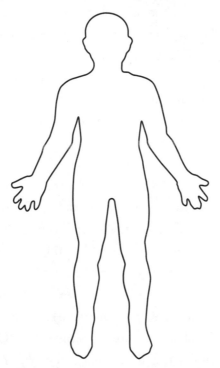

Then go back over the figure and, on top of those first words and in a different color, write what messages you felt came from your parents, i.e., *slow, fat, pretty, stupid, smart,* or *weird.* Then do the same exercise again, but this time write what messages you received in school: different color, different words. Now add in what you heard from your church (different color); your siblings (different color); husband/wife (different color); jobs (different color); your children (different color).

Once you have filled in the messages, I want you to stop and see what words are hiding underneath. How did the messages you heard growing up replace those initial ideas about who you were as a small and innocent baby? How did you allow that egocentric child to form the basis of your identity, not created from the divine self within, but through the real and perceived negative messages you heard from those around you?

For less sensitive children, the messages they received from school, home, friends, and family were all taken in stride. As they developed and matured, moving out of the egocentric stage, they were able to understand the other person's perspective, were able to take into account the environment and the circumstances in which that message might have been born. But sensitive children strap that message to themselves like a ticking bomb, living in fear of the unknown moment they are sure to detonate. Darryl was so close to his own end, he later told me, he didn't have any suicide attempts left; the next one would have been for real.

Through the work that week with his family, Darryl's mother finally stopped bringing her knitting to the group meetings. She confessed that she had felt so guilty for those years. She, too, had been overwhelmed by the change, and, not wanting to seem ungrateful, she had never shared her feelings with anyone. Once Darryl opened up the door for everyone to get honest, the family was finally able to heal. I know that I held that experience with Mr. Thompson well into my forties. One day in family therapy with my husband and children, I finally told the story I had kept underground, lurking in the dark basement of my secrets. When my own children reached out and said, "Mama, that wasn't your fault," I could finally hear the inner child within me saying the same thing. I could listen to that divine voice whispering to me, offering me the kind words I had never received from my parents. Finally I stopped living in the past, and I began to connect with that powerful present. I could feel the ground beneath my feet. And I could look in the mirror and know that I deserved all the love and joy and inspiration this world had to offer.

PART FOUR

Action

You have to know the past to understand the present.

—Dr. Carl Sagan

EIGHT

Process Prep

The founder of Alcoholics Anonymous, Bill Wilson, once wrote, "Creation gave us instincts for a purpose. . . . Yet these instincts, so necessary for our existence, often far exceed their proper functions. Powerfully, blindly, many times subtly, they drive us, dominate us, and insist upon ruling our lives."

Man was born with a God-given need for material and emotional fulfillment: craving companionship and comfort, seeking security through shelter, food, and love. From these instincts our feelings are born, as natural to human existence as air, and just as necessary. For many addicts, they do not accept these feelings as mere reactions to life, but rather as loaded concepts that they refuse to engage in, using their addictions as a shield to prevent them from experiencing emotion in a healthy manner.

Scientists have proven that emotions do not go away. As much as we try to hide, avoid, ignore them, they show up in other areas, often affecting our physical as well as emotional well-being. In Daniel Goleman's book *Emotional Intelligence,* he describes a university study wherein two women were shown films from the aftermath of Hiroshima and Nagasaki. One of the women had been given permission to express her emotional reaction to the footage, while the other was told to suppress her feelings, remaining nonchalant despite the atrocities she was viewing. Throughout the course of the film, the woman who was suppressing her feelings had increasingly higher blood pressure, her tension rising while she worked to trap her feelings inside. The study showed that having an emotional reaction to something or someone is an unstoppable, natural development of the body, and the work one must do to avoid it is far more strenuous than the work it takes to give in to the reaction.

Tamara dumped two cups of vegetables on her plate, moving slowly behind one of the other clients in her six-day. Tamara was far from obese, but with her oversize pants, baggy sweatshirts, and long dark blond hair that hung in her face, she appeared much larger than her 160-pound frame. She came to Shades because her husband was constantly complaining that she was fat. We quickly discovered that Tamara's husband was both verbally and physically abusive.

As we traditionally do at Shades, once everyone had eaten, all of the clients went around the table, standing up to offer five affirmations about what they loved about themselves, their life, and their bodies. I watched as we approached Tamara, who squirmed in her seat, barely able to focus as the other clients gave gratitude for their thighs, their stomach, the food on their plates, or their families at home. Finally it was Tamara's turn. She sighed deeply, got up, and began to mumble. She simply repeated what the others had said so she could get through this and out of the room. She stared down at her plate as she spoke.

"Tamara, look up," I interrupted her.

She stared at me as she said, "I love my hips. I love my arms."

"Really?" I asked.

"It's what you want me to say, isn't it? It's what everybody else is saying."

"Yes, but they are at least pretending to feel it. In fact, I'd wager most of them actually do. When was the last time you felt something?"

Tamara's eyes were nearly dead. "I got angry just a few minutes ago when I saw we were having fish."

"Fish? Yes, fish is annoying. Is food the only thing you get emotional about?"

Tamara stared back down at the ground. After years in an abusive relationship, she had long since lost her own voice and her own identity, let alone her right to feel. Food had become the only conduit she had for emotions, the sole arena in which she could experience joy and pain, hunger and guilt. If you want to see a food addict get angry, get in his plate. And if you really want to watch him react, ask him to share how he feels about having his food controlled by someone else. Tamara had barely spoken to anyone since her arrival, ignoring the other clients, unwilling to expose anything of her life, and now we were poking around in one of the most intimate parts of her life: her eating habits.

"Is it only food that makes you mad?" I asked Tamara as she continued to stand there, staring at the ground. She looked up at me, holding my line of vision, probably the most courageous act she had taken in some time.

"A lot makes me mad, but how can I share that? How can I tell anyone about the way I live?"

Behind Tamara's sad and lonely life hid a woman who was desperate to be in relationships with other people, to share her pain, to stand up for herself. But she was lost in her codependent and terrifying relationship. Her husband and the food were wound up in a vicious cycle that held her captive, shuffling and muttering in quiet resentment.

Feelings Aren't Facts

When Pia Mellody wrote her classic work, *Facing Codependence*, she explored how intensely our emotions factor into addiction, how "our culture divides our feelings into two kinds: 'good' and 'bad.' . . . Unfortunately, this sort of 'black or white' categorizing is erroneous and dysfunctional." Most of us have been taught that some feelings are good. Being happy, cheerful, loving are all characteristics that people are supposed to exhibit. They are signs of mature and rational behavior that are often attributed to successful relationships and general well-being. The other emotions, the "bad" feelings—shame, pain, guilt, even excessive joy— these are left to the immature, the emotional, the crazy, those folks who are not poised for adult responsibilities.

When there is any level of dysfunction in a household, a child often ends up experiencing the parents' emotions as though they were her own. She either carries those feelings for her parents or she denies them altogether. If a child has an abusive father and a codependent mother, she might take on the anger her mother didn't express, becoming enraged and even abusive herself. She will hold that anger for her mother, carrying its burden. And, not surprisingly, finding herself behaving like the parent she blames most. Or she might swing the other way. She will try to deny the feelings, focusing her time and energies on eating, shopping, or her adult relationships, believing that she can escape the cycle in which she was raised. But then one day she will blow. She will find herself screaming at her boss or her children, shocked that such rage has been boiling the whole time.

Whether we are carrying or denying those feelings from childhood, the emotion is broken off at midpoint, a tender nerve with no salve, and over time it finds its way to the surface, overtaking the person who has worked so hard, and often for many years, to keep it silenced. We fail to see the emotion as a necessary part of human existence. When we deny it, we never learn how to properly go through it. We disconnect from the feelings, and therefore whenever something happens that triggers that same emotion, we don't know what to do. So for many of us, we eat instead.

The following is a chart created by Pia Mellody. I've modified it to include "denied" feelings as well as "carried" ones. In it, you will see how these feelings get distorted and intensified from their original state. When we carry or deny them, they become destructive and unhealthy versions of the emotion in question.

FEELING	CARRIED or denied, can produce	GIFT when embraced
ANGER	*Rage*	STRENGTH ENERGY MOTIVATION
FEAR	*Panic, Paranoia*	WISDOM PROTECTION
PAIN	*Depression* *Hopelessness*	HEALING GROWTH
LONELINESS	*Isolation* *Helplessness*	REACHING IN & REACHING OUT
SHAME	*Worthlessness*	HUMILITY HUMANITY
GUILT	*Immobility*	AMENDS VALUES
JOY	*Hysteria*	HOPE HEALING SPIRITUALITY

Rather than experiencing the gifts of the feeling, the addict must suffer its most damaging consequences.

These seven emotions—anger, fear, pain, loneliness, shame, guilt, joy—are all neutral points of sentiment on their own, neither good nor bad, just the natural products of our instinctive needs. Nearly every feeling will come from those seven basic feelings. For so many food addicts, we have been disconnected from our emotions. Often, when I ask clients how they feel, they will respond with the physical manifestations of feeling: "I have a slight headache," or, "My stomach is queasy." Or they are vague about their feelings, detached and unknowing about what they feel. They will say "anxious" when really what they mean is "fearful." They end up pushing these emotions underneath their outward personas. There they fossilize into their worst aspects until the pressure gets too great and they can no longer be contained by the addictions. Those addictions are like oil derricks, drilling deeper and deeper into the carried or denied emotions. Until finally the old pockets of pain burst, gushing out across the addict's life and tearing apart whatever facade they believed would hold them in check.

But when we put a simple label to our interior emotional state, we can get in touch with those feelings. At Shades, we use these seven basic feelings to describe our mental and physical states every day. We stop complaining about our physical ailments and we look to what is going on inside: Are we angry, afraid, or lonely? When do we feel guilty and call it hunger? When do we pretend we are living in joy when really it's hysteria? And how can we stop confusing nausea with shame and headaches with emotional pain? Instead of turning to food, we evaluate what is going on inside us. We can move through it, experiencing the emotion's gift, because we finally know how to recognize and process the feeling. Recovery is about taking a problem to resolution, even if that means the whole well below the surface needs to erupt.

On Tamara's fifth day, she lost her marbles. We were all back at the table, with everyone staring down into their plates of baked chicken and creamed spinach. The room was silent, as our therapeutic work was in full swing. The clients had spent all day watching one another go through the heavy processing that this work demands. Tamara had finagled her way into going last, which meant she was the only person who had yet to do the work. Though everyone was tired, there was a sense of serenity that blanketed the table, keeping everyone quiet as they ate. That is, until Tamara's plate went flying across the room and hit the other wall. She stood up and walked outside to where one of our big oak trees stands holding two swings.

I waited a moment before following her outside.

"Well, that was something!" I called to her as she sat in one of the swings, dragging her feet in the dirt.

"I'm sorry, Mrs. McCarty," she started.

"It's Tennie, and you'd better not apologize for that."

I sat down on the swing next to her, and for a moment we sat there enjoying the brisk fall air, twilight spreading across the sky.

"I've never done anything like that before," Tamara finally said.

"Why not?"

She smiled. "Rich would kill me. Oh, my God, he wouldn't know what to do."

"It's not about Rich."

Tamara's smile fell as I continued. "You're not here for Rich, Tamara. Otherwise, he would be here. You are here for you. You are here to get the help you have always needed, to stop hiding and lying for a relationship that is only going to kill you."

I told her that we couldn't offer the help she needed in terms of the relationship and the abuse, but that if she was willing to allow herself some emotions back, she might find the strength to seek such help.

"I don't know that I have it in me, Tennie."

"Can you swing?" I asked.

She looked at me, confused.

"Because what if I told you that you've spent your whole life sitting in a swing, never realizing that it could help you to fly. Those feelings you've been hiding are what you have in you. They make up that authentic divine self. They are your strength, your courage. But as long as you're shut down, well, you'll just be dragging your feet, pretending that you don't feel."

I pushed back a little on my swing, motioning for Tamara to join me, and she did. She pumped her legs like the little girl she never really got to be, and together we went back and forth, swinging until a wonderful sound erupted from her throat: tears. Hard, powerful, angry tears. She swung and she sobbed, finally allowing those dark, painful feelings to engulf her.

Feelings are not facts, but most likely you have been treating them like they are, hiding from them as though they are a real threat to your well-being and safety. But as you move through those emotions, you will begin to recognize that those feelings are neither good nor bad, but rather gifts from God to help us grow so that we may see our most basic instincts (survival, sustenance, shelter, fellowship, love) met. You no longer need to hide from anger—use it instead as a source of motivation. Rather than turning fear into paranoia, you can have faith in the order of the universe.

But, *most important,* you can identify those feelings so that you don't confuse them with being hungry. I used to always be hungry, experiencing that physical sensation all day long. But once I was able to decipher the difference between feeling hungry and feeling an emotion I did not like, that sensation went away. I am very rarely hungry today. I know that when my emotional barometer starts telling me that I need to eat something that isn't in my meal plan, what I really need to do is look at how I am feeling. Am I ignoring some emotion that has come up? Am I carrying something for someone else? You can begin to use the food as a guide to your emotional well-being, and stop using it to control your feelings.

If It's Hysterical, It's Historical

The day after Tamara broke down on the swing set, she got up in front of the group, and though she had barely spoken a word since her arrival, she spilled every detail of her life story, from her mother's unplanned and unwanted pregnancy with her, to Tamara's marriage to a man everyone, including her parents, warned her had the "crazy" in his eyes. As Tamara described her mother's shame at getting pregnant at the age of seventeen, I stopped her. "So you felt unwanted from the start?"

Tamara immediately began stammering, "N-no, that was before they even had me. It was . . . it was just her initial reaction; she changed; she felt that . . . She . . ."

Tamara suddenly sat down, unable to breathe. It was as though the ground had just shifted and she could no longer stand. I went to her, helping her to catch her breath as she realized how those early ideas about her birth had become the foundation for her life.

I rubbed her back. "Tamara, if it's hysterical, it's historical. Your reaction right now is all the proof you need that those ideas got in; they infiltrated your life."

Anytime you experience excessive feelings about something, chances are it is because of some past event or experience that is triggering it.

This is why you must look back on your life history and see where the hysterics originated. By creating a map that marks every event that has occurred since your conception to the present, you can elucidate the patterns of emotion that underlie all of your behavior. Pull out a few sheets of paper (no more than five) and begin outlining your life from your parents' first meeting to today. For the first eighteen years, chart it out in two-year increments; from eighteen to fifty, describe every five-year period; from fifty-plus, every ten. Though everyone who does this exercise fears the amount of time and recollection it demands, there is no reason you cannot complete it within thirty minutes. Time yourself so that you focus only on the milestones of your story. Trust me, you are worth thirty minutes. If you are looking to create a new set of behaviors, relinquishing your old ones, it is going to take action on your part, and that first step starts now.

As you begin, think about what your birth was like. How was your parents' relationship at that time? Were you planned? Was there stress in your family? Describe your first years of life. What was your relationship like with your parents, and were they engaged in your upbringing? Did you have siblings, and how did you get along? Did you go to day care, and if so, what was your reaction? Were there other family members living in your home, and who were they?

What was it like when you entered grammar school? Did you enjoy it, making friends easily, or did you struggle with either its social or academic aspects? What was your home life like? What was your relationship to food during those years? When did you start noticing the opposite sex, or the same sex, and were you attracted to them? If you're a woman, at what age did you start your period?

How was your junior high/middle school experience? Were your parents involved in this part of your life? Describe your relationship with them. How did academics figure into this time in your life? Friends? Romantic relationships? What was the role of food during this period? Did you experiment with alcohol, drugs, and/or tobacco? Did you feel comfortable with yourself at this age, appreciating your body, or were you already beginning to tear it down? How did your body image affect other areas of your life, if at all?

What was life like after high school? Did you continue your education? Did you get married and/or have children? What has your role been in their upbringing? Have you suffered any sexual or emotional traumas? Describe your romantic relationships, your relationship with your parents and siblings. What has your professional life been like? What was your relationship to food during these years? Where did you overeat, binge, purge, or starve? What was going on in your life during some of your biggest food struggles?

As you have aged, how have your relationships been challenged, and where have they been healed? How have you seen food play a role in them? Have you gone through divorce, job loss, retirement? Have you passed through menopause, and what was your experience? Where are you today in your life? Physically? Financially? Romantically? Professionally? Emotionally?

Everything should be included in this life map—secrets, things you don't discuss with others. This is your life story.

Once you have completed your life map, writing everything out, set it aside. In the next chapter, you will be reviewing that life history to identify where and how those seven basic emotions have occurred throughout your life. You will see where those feelings became their most destructive aspects (where anger became rage, loneliness turned into isolation), and later we will look at how you can transform those feelings into their gifts. We will see where anger can be motivating, and where loneliness is a sign to reach into yourself and out to others.

We will be using your seven different-colored pens to highlight where these seven basic emotions have shown up in your life. You will be reviewing your life story and marking where the emotion has arisen with its assigned color. You can use your red pen to highlight anger, green for fear, black for pain, yellow for loneliness, blue for shame, orange for guilt, and purple to acknowledge joy; or mix them up however you choose. Any eight-pack of markers should work just fine. By the time you are finished, your history should look like a rainbow.

After Tamara's stay with us, she moved over to a women's shelter that treats women suffering from domestic abuse. She was finally strong enough to free herself from the abusive and addictive cycles in which she had lived. Not along ago, she wrote me, "There was so much inside me that I failed to see. I didn't know what I was capable of so I just shut down. I have so much strength in me when I am willing to access it." As do you.

NINE

Processing Our Feelings

*I*f we have nothing else, we have our stories. Those histories anchor us to reality, to every moment lived, every pain endured, the hardships and joys that make up our human experience. For many folks, they have lived their whole lives removed from this story, ignorant of its role in their present. But when we look back at what has happened, we can begin to integrate new behaviors into our lives.

Addictions are a disease of the feelings. For most addicts, it is not anyone else's behavior that sends them back into the dependency; it is their own. They make poor choices, responding to life in an unhealthy manner, knowing that a substance or process will take them out of those feelings, and so the cycle continues. They ignore their histories, deny or carry the feelings, using food, avoiding food, and going shopping so they don't have to be present. And it works.

I could hear Scott's car coming from a mile away once he finally arrived at Shades. After months of discussions with his cardiologist, his therapist, his personal assistant, and a bevy of other doctors and enablers, Scott decided he needed more help than his team of aides could offer. At more than four hundred pounds, he was a human vacuum—consuming food, women, alcohol, drugs, anything that stood in his path. His eating was out of control, but his spending was what had really begun to take a toll on his life. For as much money as Scott made as a big-time screenwriter, he had also been incurring enormous debt. He was on the verge of bankruptcy—physical, financial, and spiritual.

After renting a Mercedes convertible in Abilene, he raced his way through Buffalo Gap, screeching to a halt outside of the administrative building. He told Cam that he could stay for only four days, but after she explained that we couldn't admit him for less than the full week, he agreed to stay for the six-day intensive program. If we thought his tantrum over not being able to drive his newly rented car was bad, we were nowhere near prepared for his reaction to having his phone, pills, and iPad confiscated. He threw his suitcase, screamed at one of our staff, and then ripped up the first book handed to him that outlined his week at Shades. The staff member left the room, leaving him to sit and sulk. Finally Scott calmed down and quickly apologized to everyone.

Over the next few days, we watched addiction in action. Scott was like a child who had been using food and anything money could buy (not to mention drugs and alcohol) to manage life, and in turn, he never grew up. He didn't know how to process the most basic of emotions. Anger turned into violent screaming almost immediately. Pain overtook him in racking sobs that no one could control. Even joy was hysterical, so loud and visceral that he was not allowed to hug anyone for fear of knocking them over.

When he finally stood up to read his life history to the group, I could feel his persona growing, as though he were preparing for a dramatic monologue.

"Stop," I said before he could even begin. "I want you to do this a little differently. I want you to kneel down and whisper your story. Say it as though it is an intimate prayer, not something to be dramatized or glorified, but something to be revered."

"You didn't ask anyone else to do that," Scott rebutted, folding his arms.

"I know, Scott. But I don't want you to not feel this, to use your personality as a defense mechanism. We can't solve our problems unless we are willing to look at how they make us feel, until we stop and ask, 'Just what is the real problem here?' Once we stop using the food, the feelings will come out, and they are not the feelings of the grown-up in charge—they are the feelings of the child who was not allowed to process them in the first place. I want your adult to come on board for this, to take it seriously. And yes, it's different from what the others did, but haven't you been telling us this whole time that you're different?"

When we are in our addictions, we act like children. Physically—and financially—we may play the role of grown-ups, but our emotional responses are so underdeveloped, we don't know how to react when something triggers those oft-denied emotions. Recovery from addiction is about growing up.

That day, as Scott knelt on the ground, whispering his story, weeping quietly, he was able to see all the emotions he had been ignoring, shouting over, eating, and living like a glutton to avoid. And he began to experience them. Finding the quiet in his own storm, he could see where all seven of those primary emotions—anger, pain, fear, loneliness, shame, guilt, and joy—had a rightful place in life. And through the process of recovery, he understood his story. Writing and rewriting its narrative, he established his foundation for the future.

Anger

Throughout the course of mankind, nearly every great movement has been born out of anger. Many leaders see injustice and they are infuriated by it, motivating them to create change. That is anger's healthy use, which we all have a right to, allowing it to inspire us to grow, to provoke, to demand that things be different so that they may be better. Nelson Mandela once said, "When the water starts boiling it is foolish to turn off the heat." And so with anger, it is not an emotion to be turned off halfway, but rather one to be harnessed for good, for the benefit of one's life and the world at large.

When Olympians are preparing for a race, they might train with friends, colleagues, relatives, people whom they like and even love. But when it's time for competition, they need to have some anger in them, engaging that fire to let them run faster than the person next to them. If this athlete is emotionally healthy, once the race ends—win, lose, or draw—the anger is gone. Though he might be upset or disappointed, he will focus on what he could have done differently, how he might prepare in the future, but not on the person who won. However, if that competitor isn't healthy, he will hold on to that anger. He will find himself at a bar twenty years later, yelling at a rerun of the race on TV, blaming his competitor for the loss.

Instead of processing the anger, using it as a force for change, a guide to what they might do differently in their lives, food addicts will often force the anger down, allowing it to fester into resentment. Over the years, they blame those resentments for their behaviors, believing that they are the cause of all of life's challenges. And life is challenging—for all of us. We see injustices at work, in our family, in the parking lot, and on TV, and are aware that the world is filled with cruel events and unfair acts. And it is human to be incensed by this. But, sadly, many of us have been raised to think that anger isn't good, and, because of this, we do not know how to process the emotion in a healthy way. We stand there holding that hot coal of rage, not knowing where to throw it or how to let it go, burning our hands instead. And then we look around at our husband, our mother, our children, and we scream, "You made me do this! It's all your fault." We are blind to the role we have played in our own self-injury. Though indeed others might have done us harm, we have long lost the opportunity to confront them in an honest and productive fashion. Instead we lash out at them because we failed to take the right action in the first place.

When Jamie maxed out her last credit card, she knew she had a problem. A forty-five-year-old therapist from Manhattan, she spent every day listening to the woes of others, and then returning home to the apartment she shared with her abusive and controlling mother. Jamie had been battling her weight all her life, but once she began to make some money, a new addiction emerged: shopping. As long as she had the right clothes, the perfectly crafted exterior, Jamie was able to ignore the weight, and she did her best to ignore the abusive woman living in her home. But after years of hiding behind an increasingly expensive and depressing mask, Jamie became exhausted. One night she lost it, turning on her mother. She threatened that she was going to hurt them both if the old woman didn't stop nagging her. A week later, she entered herself in our six-week residential program, ready for help. On her first day, she sat down with me, explaining:

> It's almost like the anger turns into self-pity and then the self-pity turns into anger, and it's such a vicious cycle. I see anger show up in my self-destructive tendencies and in my self-entitlement, where I think people owe me things. I don't tell them that, but then when they don't do what

I think they ought to do, I become enraged. Because I haven't accepted or dealt with my anger, the resentment builds and it squelches my spirit, my zest for life.

Despite a childhood filled with abuse and abandonment, Jamie had used her anger for motivation, completing college and receiving her master's degree, becoming quite successful. But when it came to her personal life, she did not know how to use that anger to change the relationship with her mother, or how to begin creating more boundaries within her life. With no healthy direction for her anger to flow, Jamie just kept taking her mother's abuse, swallowing her criticisms and negativity, trying to play the role of the good daughter, all while the rage boiled within.

For others, it is not their own anger with which they are dealing, but the frustrations they incur when watching injustice done to someone else. They take on that fury for their parents, siblings, or even neighbors, because that other person is incapable of managing anger themselves. By the time I left my mother's house, I had spent decades swallowing the bitter pills of my mother's denial. She had always responded to my father's violence with self-medication, never learning to process her own anger. Though my mother would scream at my father, she never stood up for herself in a true and powerful way. And in the end, she was always the one left broken. I just felt so bad for that woman, incensed at how my father treated her, indignant that she was always so alone. Then, as I grew up, I turned that emotion inward, literally carrying it in my belly.

Over time, that vile little monster that lived within turned from anger to rage, and I would go from being "sweet Tennie," pouring lemonade and baking pies, into this vicious witch everyone would work to stay clear of. I would lie in bed at night, waiting for RL to come home, knowing he was out drinking, the anger in me building. Finally he would teeter into the bedroom, trying to be quiet but creating a drunken tornado in his wake before falling into bed. The whole time, I would pretend to sleep, thinking of how easy it would be to take the pillow and smother his face. The rage consuming me, I would imagine his feet kicking as he tried to struggle against my weight, and the freedom that would come from knowing that I would never have to wait for his sorry ass to stumble home again. I could feel that rage in me brewing, that desire to strike out so that other people could feel it, too. I could taste the shock and horror that I would have felt if I had done the deed. Though I never actually attempted murder (thank God!), I would still find myself saying and doing things I could never take back.

For so many folks who struggle with food, the anger is kept calm by the mashed potatoes, the large pizza, and the Girl Scout cookies. This is even more the case for eating-disorder folks than it is with other addicts, who use alcohol or drugs to lower their inhibitions, allowing them moments when they are able to express their anger. But for food addicts, often the only thing that will get them to express their anger is to mess with their food.

By her second week Jamie, the well-educated, self-aware psychologist, had stopped talking altogether. Though her hair was still perfectly in place, the shoes matching the belt and scarf, the anger she had been managing through food was just oozing from her pores. Her "lookism"— shopping for the perfect outfits, spending money she didn't have on shoes whose labels made them cost too much—had been her shield as much as the food. Jamie needed to be in control. It was how she managed those feelings that were boiling inside her. And now that we controlled the menu, she rebelled.

She didn't want to eat the healthy food, demanding cheeseburgers and french fries, bristling at being forced to eat on our schedule, and filled with enough anger to explode Buffalo Gap.

After one of our group sessions, she came up to me. "I want to call my mother."

"Okay, well, you have phone time tomorrow morning, right?"

"This isn't prison, Tennie. I want to call her now." The anger I saw flash in her eyes I had seen in my own. There is nothing like telling a control freak that she has no control.

I just nodded. "Well, I have an idea. We can get you on the phone with her now, but I think that means you're going to have to spend a few days looking a little more natural." She stared at me as I continued. "No makeup, you'll wear your pajamas, no matching."

"You can't do that!" She screamed in my face, getting close to me.

"Jamie, you can leave here whenever you want, but unless you're willing to do anything, try anything to get better, you're just gonna return to the same old mess. I know you're smart. You've got this all figured out. But having it in your head won't mean much until you connect it with your heart, until you start responding with love instead of reacting in anger. Do you want to try to release some of that?"

At Shades, we use a form of experiential therapy in which patients beat up a large beanbag square with a padded bat, letting go of all that rage they have pent up inside. Experiential therapy allows people to engage their senses. Instead of just talking about their troubles, they use their sight, their touch, and their energy to communicate those feelings. We use the beanbag for a lot of anger and shame therapy, where people often have trouble voicing those emotions. They are better able to release them through their bodies by using safe force and pressure to allow the feelings a way to come out. When I asked Jamie if she wanted to try it, she nodded slowly as my daughter Kim went and got the bag.

"Honey, you're not going to change until you let go of all those old behaviors, and I don't just mean the food. It's the rage that's killing you, that's eating you up like a cancer."

We handed Jamie the bat and began to have her describe how her mother treated her. We asked her to get that anger at her mother out, taking it to the bag instead of holding it in. Jamie was quiet at first, but

Kim and I kept pressing her. "Tell her you have the right to be angry, that you are giving her back your anger."

As Jamie began to repeat the words, she got louder, the bat slamming down harder; she began screaming and yelling as the rage took over, finally finding a safe place to expose itself. By the time she was finished, Jamie was slumped over. I went and held her, and she curled up in my arms like a little girl. I asked her how she felt, and she smiled through her tears. "I don't feel hungry."

Finally Jamie started participating in mealtime, eating the food offered, and not making requests she knew would be denied. Over the next few days, she was also stripped of her other survival techniques: her perfectly matched clothes, the ballet flats, and the coiffed hair. She would silently cry while eating the food in front of her, accepting healthy choices for the first time in her life. As hard as it was for her to do, she was finally opening herself up to the emotions that she had trapped inside. It wasn't about the food; it was about her need to manipulate everything around her through those triplets of addiction—by eating, by shopping, and by staying in the codependent relationship with her mother. She was finally letting it go, releasing all that emotion that had been festering underneath her sweet smiles and intelligent insights.

Confronting Anger

Now go ahead and look back at your life map. Take out one of your colored markers—whichever you have decided to use for anger—and read through your story.

Think back to when you were that original divine child, and remember when you began to hold these feelings of anger. At what age? Where did you suppress that anger, and how has it been expressed as its negative manifestation, rage? As you look through your life map, where have you been enraged, violent, saying or doing things you didn't want to do or were ashamed by later?

Do you see in your life map where you learned to deny anger? Were there points when you carried that anger for a parent, a sibling, a relative? Are there patterns in your family dynamic where its suppression has turned to rage? How has that affected your family? How has it affected you? Do you see where the rage has altered your own life and relationships?

Take some time with this work—don't get up and get any food to make it go away. Sit in the feelings of anger. Allow yourself to cry, yell, scream if you have to. Go through the process. Take a walk or do some jumping jacks; allow the rage to leave your body in a healthy way. Feel what it's like to process this emotion as opposed to letting it control you. Allowing it to run through your nervous system, feel it pumping from your heart through your arms, your legs. Allow it to flow through your stomach and mind, passing quickly through your body and emptying out through the top of your head, the palms of your hands, and the bottoms of your feet.

Anger is a completely healthy emotion, one we all have a right to. Love yourself for being angry, saying out loud, "I have the right to be angry."

If you want to think about whom you are angry at, you can address those words to them as though they are there: "Mother, I have a right to be angry at you"; "Husband, I have a right to be angry at you"; "Wife, I have a right to be angry at you"; "Father, I have a right to be angry at you"; "Child, I have a right to be angry at you."

Feel what it is like to find your voice again. Many people suffering from food addiction have lost that voice. They stuff that anger down, keeping quiet about the injustices they have seen in their own lives and in the world around them, and it eats them up alive. Get it out! The anger, the rage. Get it all out.

Fear

I count my lucky stars every day to be blessed with the feeling of fear. As with our other emotions, God gave us healthy fear as a means of protection. It tells us to get out of the burning house. It says, "Don't pull the car into traffic." It teaches us not to put ourselves in positions of harm, preventing us from walking down the dark alley or jumping off the balcony. But unhealthy fear teaches us to be afraid of things even if they are not a threat.

Instead of protecting us, fear becomes "False Evidence Appearing Real." We begin to live in panic and paranoia, because we know that the other shoe is always preparing to drop. We believe the world is an unsafe place bent on disappointing us, and the universe is a cruel lover—offering us care and protection and pulling out the rug just as we finally relax. We figure, *Well, if that's how God is going to treat me, why should I have faith? Faith in what?*

Addicts can get just a smidgen of this false evidence and decide that the worst-case scenario is inevitable, building that case against the universe and themselves. If a normal person is on the highway and gets a flat, he will call AAA. If an addict gets one, he will call the suicide hotline. Addicts do not believe that things are going to work out, thinking that every negative occurrence speaks to some great trauma or tragedy they have suffered or will soon suffer. They become like Henny Penny—"The sky is falling, the sky is falling!"—bringing that negativity into the life of everyone around them. Their doubt runs so deep, they are not able to believe in anything, retreating further into paranoia, and losing sight of all the glory and possibility this magnificent world contains once we allow ourselves to trust in it.

For Scott, our successful screenwriter, fear had been the foundation of his childhood, as both of his parents had lost family in the Holocaust.

After Scott completed the six-day intensive program, we recommended that he stay for the six-week residential program. Though at first he was convinced that his whole career would go down the toilet if he was gone from it that long, he had begun to experience a change, a shift in his psyche that he couldn't understand, but felt might be related to the work we were doing at Shades. Finally, it came time for his Family Week, his mother and father flying in from New York to participate, a bold act for both of them, as they rarely left their neighborhood. During the family sculpt, other clients played the role of Scott's parents, who were so afraid of the world outside their front door, they wouldn't even take their only child to the movies. The client playing Scott's father replayed the conversation that echoed throughout his childhood: "There won't be enough parking," to which the client acting as his mother replied, "We'll never be able to get good seats." The fears progressed as the parents tried to keep Scott inside. In elementary and middle school, they wouldn't allow him to participate in sports or play out on the streets with other neighborhood children. Later, they begged him not to go to Los Angeles for school, though he was offered a full scholarship, and badgered him about coming home to work in the family business, which was a much safer choice than Hollywood. They lived in panic and paranoia, and they passed them along to Scott.

He finally broke down in front of them. "I don't trust anything or anyone. I am always so scared that people are out to cheat me, I don't even know how to love; all I know how to do is control, because if I'm giving you money, then you're mine and you can't hurt me."

He turned to his parents. "All of this, everything I have done, is to prove you wrong, to show you I could do it, because I thought you didn't believe in me. But now I see it: You don't believe in anything, and I'm exactly the same way."

He sat down on the ground, his voice quiet. "I want to believe in something."

People often say that the opposite of faith is fear. This doesn't mean that we make irrational decisions and wait for God to fix them; rather, when we take the next right action and ask for God's help, we have little to fear. We are able to reach out to others, to make friends, and to believe in a world we can trust.

Children's nervous systems are so highly tuned, able to perceive the fears and pains suffered by their parents that the children often adopt those emotions as their own once they move into adulthood. For Scott, it wasn't until he found recovery that he could recognize this, looking at his family history and realizing his fear was nothing but an instinct that had been stretched far beyond its purpose. Though his parents had received that message of fear from family who had experienced some of the most significant and real trauma in history, that extreme need to protect was unnecessary in the world in which they raised Scott. Where fear should have been a healthy warning, it forced him and his family inside, isolating Scott from friends, sports, and all the normal activities of growing up, instead ensnaring him in a lifetime of food addiction.

Scott confessed that at age six, he started binge-eating whenever his parents weren't around, eating from a storage cellar in the basement, the pantry, and the cookie jar. He didn't have any friends, but he had food, and it numbed him; it made him feel safe. His parents had tried desperately to do the same thing—to keep him at home, away from the dangers of childhood and life. But instead of security, they offered him paranoia. They taught him through their own carried fears that the world was a terrible place with untrustworthy people. They didn't mean to isolate their only child, but that was the natural effect of their behaviors. Scott grew up in loneliness, and found food to be his only comfort. Once he was old enough, he swung to the opposite side of the pendulum—risking his life through his behaviors as a rejection of his parents' belief system.

When we work through a client's fears, we help him see reality. We ask him to look at where that fear is coming from. Is there an immediate danger? Is it a life-or-death situation (and very few things are)? More often than not, it has little to do with the present, rooted instead in the messages of a client's past.

Scott told me later, "I've been such a fearful person, terrified of other people, and just hiding out behind all my things. But once I began to recover, to get a community around me, I realized that the fear wasn't going to hurt me unless I let it. That false evidence was only that . . . false. It was up to me to decide what was going to be real in my life, whether I was going to live free of those fears or be chained to them. I started working on the fear, and it felt like I was working toward being whole. It's called healing."

Uncovering Fear

As you review your life map, take another colored marker and highlight where fear has taken place in your life. When were you afraid? What made you feel this way? Were your parents afraid? When did you start believing that you weren't being taken care of? And where in your life have you made choices or decisions based on fear, recognizing where you were wrong or manipulative because you were afraid your needs would not be met?

There are a million forms of fear. Fear can resemble insecurity, or it can appear as overconfidence. People can be paralyzed by fear, or they can make rash decisions because of it. Fear can come out in so many ways, dressed up as another emotion altogether, resembling anger, shame, even joy. We can mask our fear by acting as though nothing is wrong, pretending that we are happy and carefree, when really we are ignoring the real or false threats that are posed in our life. As you examine your life map, how have you disguised fear? Where have you mistaken fear as inability? As insecurity? Where has it affected your self-esteem? Your personal relationships? Your material or emotional security? When has fear eroded important things in your life: jobs, relationships, and ambitions?

As you identify the times you have acted out of panic or paranoia, what has your behavior looked like? Did you act arrogant to hide insecurities? Did you hurt someone else because you were afraid to be hurt? Set aside the wrongs done by others, and highlight where you have been selfish because of fear. Where have you been dishonest? Self-seeking?

When our parents teach us how to deny or carry our feelings, that is exactly what we are going to teach our children, passing it along and watching as the next generation reacts much the same way, believing that false evidence to be real.

Pain

Deirdre arrived at Shades of Hope in a wheelchair, sick from years of drinking castor oil (a laxative best used in small amounts). She sat in my office, staring out at the large oak tree that embraces the main courtyard at Shades. At the age of twenty-six, she was curled over like an old woman suffering from osteoporosis, and when I asked her what brought her to Shades of Hope, I had to lean in close to even hear her quiet and defeated voice. She softly replied, "I just can't keep moving. I know I am going to die, and though I hurt so bad, I don't want to; I just want the pain to go away."

Deirdre had been working her way through college, taking care of her two little sisters, until she got so sick she could do none of it. Deirdre had a childhood that no one should suffer. After her father committed suicide, she was abandoned by her mother and left alone to raise her siblings at the age of sixteen. They hid from social services, squatting in buildings to make do. As a child she had experienced significant sexual and physical abuse, but had used her anger to get through school, to work a full-time job . . . to just keep moving. When she came to us, she was a frightened, angry mess, but she knew she needed help. Though she had little money, we worked out a system where she could afford our care. She would have surely died without it.

On that first morning, she told me she had been drinking a bottle of castor oil every day. On its own, castor oil is an old-time laxative, but Deirdre was taking it way past its daily allowance, turning it into a poison. And she was violently ill because of it. She later shared, "When I came to Shades, I was in so much pain. I had gone through years of abuse, and then I put myself through more years of abuse. I didn't think I would ever heal. I didn't know I could."

Lance Armstrong once said, "Pain is temporary. It may last a minute, or an hour, or a day, or a year, but eventually it will subside and something else will take its place. If I quit, however, it lasts forever." For so many addicts, they quit halfway, refusing that pain-body its completion. It continues to live within them, a cancer growing in their psyche, metastasizing over the years until they get so sick from the food, the relationships, their own behaviors, that they are overcome with it. They suffer depression, anxiety, and a sense of hopelessness that leads many to believe that there is no way out.

For a lot of us food addicts, we think that emotional pain can kill us. And sometimes it can, driving us to hurt ourselves, to contemplate, attempt, and even commit suicide. The pain becomes too much, the despair too thick, and we are no longer able to see the light. We become trapped in that dark well in which we have climbed down trying to hide from the experiences and hurt we didn't know how to feel.

Not everyone who comes to Shades has attempted suicide, but even if they haven't had plans, most people have had the thought. When eating doesn't work anymore—when the outside substances or processes can't make the pain go away—they think that if only they could leave, the feelings would go with them. They want so badly to return to the light, they think the only way out is to walk into it.

Unfortunately, for many addicts, pain and depression are inextricably linked. Unable to confront the pain, folks find themselves suffering depression's classic symptoms: listlessness, an inability to get out of bed, suicidal thoughts, and a deeply penetrating sense of woe. They take pills. They might even make it to a therapist, but the depression clings. They still feel either numb or detached from life, living in that depression, all while believing that life is fair only if there is no discomfort. For some, they battle real and chronic depression or other mental illnesses. But for many others, their depression is a natural and inevitable companion to their addictions. And for those latter folks, they have a choice: either stay in the pain, or walk through it.

A dear friend once told me, "When you're going through hell, don't stop." Pain is nothing more than the most guaranteed part of existence, and ironically, it is also one of our greatest teachers. It offers us the opportunity to grow, and forces us to heal, to see where we need to change our behaviors. To paraphrase Proust, to goodness and hope we make promises, but pain we obey. Either we continue bingeing, purging, restricting, begging others to love us, or we get tired of the disease and decide to do something about it.

Deirdre had so many unresolved feelings on the inside, and had sat in that depression and hopelessness for so long, she had taken her addiction to the absolute max. She was driving herself into her own confinement and was unable to escape. She knew she would either die hiding from the pain or she would survive by feeling it. She chose to feel.

After her first month at Shades, Deirdre began to open up to the other clients. One day in our group session she shared, "I used to brag about the fact that I hadn't cried in a year. I always took care of everything, and I was always taking care of people, but I didn't let myself feel.

I would think, 'Oh, God, just get over it.' But I have learned that when we allow the pain to pass, we grow spiritually."

She was already out of her wheelchair at that time, and though she was still weak, I could see her gaining strength, both physically and emotionally. She recently celebrated two years abstinent from bulimia, and at the dinner to celebrate, I leaned over and asked her, "You still brag about not crying?"

She shook her head no. "Sometimes I have an emotion come up, and I'll cry like a child for an hour. I will be sobbing. Then, when I stop, it's like a brand-new day. It feels cleansing, and it feels good."

When we go through that pain, we are then able to reach out to others and share the experience of how we made it through. Every time I am walking through something I don't like or something that hurts, I ask myself, *Where is the lesson here? And how can this experience help someone else?*

Thanks to the fellowship of twelve-step programs, you never have to walk through anything alone again. Unfortunately, this makes it a lot harder to live in self-pity. We can no longer cry and moan that our suffering is unique. Spend any time in a meeting of Overeaters Anonymous or Anorexics and Bulimics Anonymous and you will quickly see that you are not alone. Folks have harder and easier stories, but they all have stories. And suddenly, that great wallow of self-pity begins to look a little thin. Thank God, because there is nothing more dangerous for an addict than self-pity. Once we start obsessing about how terrible our lives are, we cry, "Poor me, poor me, pour me a milk shake." We stop searching for the solution, and instead lose ourselves to the problem.

PROCESSING PAIN

Pain is a fact. If I cut my hand, it will hurt, but it is up to me how quickly and effectively I want to heal, depending on how I treat the wound. It is how we deal with pain that determines its consequences, either sinking us into depression and hopelessness, or helping us to grow. For most of us, we will find ourselves at the bottom of that pit alone, confused, and we will look up and think there is no way out—but there is. Today you can take that first step by recognizing where that pain originates.

Evaluate your life map, pulling out one of your colored pens or markers (whichever you have chosen to highlight pain), and identify where pain has shown up in your life. How has it caused depression or that sense of hopelessness? When have you tried to ignore the pain, discounting events in your life and their significance? Did something happen in your childhood? Any abuse, a divorce, physical or emotional abandonment, an unreliable parent figure and/or a traumatic experience that you have minimized so as not to feel? When have you carried pain for others, seeing it in your family, holding it as though it were yours? Were there times when you had thoughts of suicide? Did you participate in self-harm, i.e., cutting or burning yourself? Did you binge-drink, take drugs, or act recklessly? Highlight the periods in your life with your marker when the pain became too much or you had to use food or other substances to manage it.

When have you suffered from depression? Have you ever treated it through therapy or medication? When in your life did the depression or hopelessness become more severe, showing up in your sleeping patterns, your behaviors at home, in school, at work? Can you identify a manic cycle in your life—times when you experienced extreme joy, even hysteria, and other times when it felt like you would never get out of bed again?

Look back at the most painful parts of your life story, and give yourself the gift of feeling what that experience was like. Feel the hurt, the betrayal, the fear, and the terror; invite them in, holding on to that child who went through it all. Cradle yourself with the love this pain has deserved all along. Go ahead and cry. Just like Deirdre does now, cry like a little child; feel that pain sweep over you, moving through your system; cry it all out. If you need to set a time limit for yourself to feel safer, do so. Give yourself fifteen or thirty minutes just to lie there and sob, and then when you are finished, go outside, open up the curtains, and allow the world's natural light to shine on your face.

Loneliness

Companionship and solitude are key to the human experience, both of which are loved and despised by most people with equal tenacity. For most food addicts, however, they cannot appreciate either, yearning to relate to others, yet only further segregating themselves through their addiction.

The novelist Thomas Wolfe once wrote, "The whole conviction of my life now rests upon the belief that loneliness, far from being a rare and curious phenomenon, peculiar to myself and to a few other solitary men, is the central and inevitable fact of human existence." Sadly, most of us still think that this statement applies only to us addicts; believing that we are terminally unique, we reject the fellowship of others even when it is presented to us.

We engage with food, dancing with it as though it is a lover. We turn our life and will over to its consolation, ignorant or incapable of being in a true relationship to anyone or anything else.

When I was eight, my mother started taking care of a terminally ill woman who was married to a judge in Midland. For years the elderly couple lived in this lonely old two-story house with a rotting wood frame and high Victorian peaks. My mother would bring me there after school, and I would get lost in the place. Hiding in old cedar closets, their claw-footed bathtubs, I would pretend that the house was all mine.

For weeks, I had been curious about the scents that were emanating from the kitchen, knowing that the family had a cook, like most wealthy folks at that time. Finally I decided to go in there and meet her, even though I could barely speak around strangers.

"Well, hello, baby" were Hazel's first words to me. A large black woman who spent her days and nights fixing meals for the strange couple, and cleaning the old house, Hazel became one of my first and only friends. Over the next few months, I started spending more time in her kitchen than I did alone, forsaking the guest bathroom tub for her warm and kind companionship. She would ask me about school and boys, and I even began to reach out a bit, finding out that she had four children and ten grandchildren of her own. I remember telling her that one day I would have ten grandchildren, too (today I'm halfway there!), as I helped her whisk the eggs for one of the wonderful cakes Hazel would make the judge nearly every day. I would stand and help her smooth that thick and creamy frosting across the top of the cooling cake, the aroma tickling my nose. My stomach would groan to the point where Hazel would start to laugh.

It was one of the greatest times of my life. I can still hear the pots and pans banging, see the sugar sitting out on the countertop, and hear Hazel's voice echoing through the kitchen, bringing to life that lonely house and my even lonelier childhood. One day Hazel made the judge this incredible banana bread with vanilla frosting. It was perfect, just the right size, with a white cap of sweet buttercream smoothed into a wave. I loved food the way most folks love other people: with a flush in my heart, a blush on my cheeks, and the twinkle of euphoria in my eyes. And that day, after Hazel left work early to help her daughter move, I just couldn't hold back. My mother was upstairs. She barely came down to check on me anymore now that I had found a friend in Hazel. I knew that I had at least an hour before the judge came home expecting to find his cake.

I lifted up the aluminum cover to that bread as if I were getting into bed with someone, nervous and excited with anticipation. I didn't even grab a fork, my little hands digging in, consuming it with all the passion of an eight-year-old heart.

As soon as I was finished, I realized that the judge would wonder where his dessert was for the day. I knew he would get mad at Hazel for leaving early, presumably forgetting to make his own substitution for love (because at his size, he was probably finding the same solace in her cakes). I hid the evidence of my betrayal, throwing away the tin in which the cake had been made. I begged my mama for us to leave so I could get home, the cake turning in my stomach now feeling like a terrible mistake. I couldn't believe I had betrayed my only friend, choosing food over her kindness. The next day I heard the judge berate her, but she never told him what happened, taking the brunt of it for me. After that, I stopped spending time in Hazel's kitchen, retreating to the claw-footed bathtub upstairs. I remember at one point Hazel telling me that as long as I kept my fingers to myself, I could come back, but I didn't believe that I would be able to keep such a promise. Over the years, my guilt and shame over my behaviors would lose me a number of friends. I wouldn't know how to apologize or make the situation right, so instead I would hide from people who had tried to befriend me. I would back out of whatever relationship had been offered, believing I didn't deserve it. Shutting down, I would be consumed by that total empty aloneness as I became helpless against my behaviors.

Food addicts get comfortable being with food. It speaks our language and is always there, not asking for us to show up, forgiving all indiscretions. And isolation works perfectly. We don't have to deal with other people, don't have to put ourselves on the line. We just hide in our rooms like children and ignore the rest of the world until, ultimately, the world comes knocking, and we must decide whether we are going to answer.

Giving up that relationship to food means that we have to step up to the plate and be with people. We must reach inside to the God of our understanding and reach out to another human being, finding the place where we are not alone or terminally unique. Instead, we create a new camaraderie with folks who have been where we have been and who can appreciate those trials. As we find more people who share our experience, we can begin to reach out to those who might not: our family, our friends. We offer them the lessons we have learned from recovery, bringing healing and compassion into all of our affairs. We can love and appreciate companionship and loneliness, not finding the pain in either, but rather the growth.

LONELINESS DISCOVERED

Loneliness was such a commonplace experience for me, I didn't even realize how pervasive it was in my life. While I was raising seven children in a blended household, I would have never considered myself lonely, but later, when I looked back on those years, I realized they were some of the most isolated and helpless years of my life. I was utterly alone amid a sea of people. As you look at your life map, choose another pen and begin to mark where you have experienced loneliness in your life. Where in your childhood were you alone? As a teenager? As an adult? Did you carry this loneliness for someone else? Your mother? Your father?

Notice when this feeling of loneliness turned into isolation. When have you pushed others away because of it? When have you lost out on opportunities or experiences because you didn't want to engage with others? Where have you felt isolated even within a large group of family, friends, or business associates? And where have you alienated people in order to be alone?

Where did your loneliness make you feel helpless? Were there times in your life when it felt like nobody understood you? That you had nowhere to turn? Take a look at where food has played a part in this isolation. When have you chosen food over other people? Can you see the periods in your life when you turned to food for comfort? When did it begin, and how has it progressed?

For too long, we have equated loneliness with hunger, and companionship with food, believing that as long as we are full, we are content. But as you reflect back on your life and behaviors, see where true loneliness occurred, that deep and isolated place to which food was merely a passing relief. As you continue through this work, observe how that hunger takes place when you are alone. Ask yourself whether you want for food or for companionship. Watch the behavior, and allow yourself to sit in the loneliness. Use this time as an opportunity for reflection, meditation, deeper thought, and see where you can start breaking down the diseased relationship with food.

Shame

There are two different kinds of shame in this world: healthy shame and toxic shame. Healthy shame says we're all alike, like the pebble on the beach. It teaches us that we are each a child of God—absolutely perfect, and absolutely human. As Pia Mellody once described, healthy shame is when you're staying in the house with a bunch of people and you go in the bathroom and you do your business. The smell of your own waste doesn't bother you; you're used to it. But then you leave the bathroom and someone else walks in and says, "Ewww, it smells in here." We get a little embarrassed by our humanness. If we didn't, we'd be so up on the pedestal we'd think our waste didn't stink. Knowing it does is normal healthy human shame.

Toxic shame is caused by abuse: physical, emotional, psychological, spiritual, mental, and other. There is sexual abuse, which can be overt and covert. Overt is when a child is touched or forced to participate in sexual acts. Covert is when a child is exposed to anything that is not age-appropriate, i.e., pornography, sexual conversations, and explicit behaviors. We often see a lot of intellectual abuse in which the child is told she is stupid or is treated as though she doesn't know anything.

In all of these types of abuse, the character of the child is attacked. As Pia Mellody explains in *Facing Codependence*, "[W]hen a caregiver abuses a child, the caregiver is out of touch with his or her own healthy shame. . . . If the caregiver could feel healthy shame, he or she would stop abusing the child. As a result of being abused by a shameless parent . . . the child somehow develops a core of shame induced by the parent during abuse, which causes the child to feel worthless."

Our value as human beings is forever linked with how we process and experience shame. For those who have suffered its unhealthy version, who have been abused in some way in their childhood or even as adults, the shame negates their value. It teaches them that they do not merit the same rights and privileges as other humans. This often comes from their caregivers or other adults in their childhood who, through their own behaviors, passed along a message that the child was not worthy of respect or love.

A day in the life of a child is much different from a day in the life of an adult. A child's self-centeredness filters everything through this concept of good and bad. If a child is loved, nurtured, offered the respect and attentiveness that he so deserves, he will most likely grow up believing that he has a fair and inalienable place in this world. However, if he is abused in some way, that value system will be so distorted, he will believe that he is at fault, guilty of the crimes committed against him.

Andrea sat across the room from her parents, curled up into a ball. Though it was the third day of Family Week, she was still refusing to speak. Angered that she had been sent here, Andrea had been shut down since her arrival, walking with her shoulders slumped and an attitude so defiant even our staff had to take deep breaths around her. Though she looked like a little doll, with long black hair and porcelain white skin, she had been in and out of prison for years, battling drug addiction, which was often supported through prostitution. After years of living in different states, Andrea had finally returned home and asked her parents for help. Andrea's parents took one look at her emaciated frame and worried that Andrea's problems were more than drugs. They took her to a doctor and realized she was also battling severe bulimia and anorexia. Though Andrea was hoping that her parents would respond to her appeal for help with a car and some money, she found herself on a plane to Buffalo Gap, pissed off and refusing to participate.

Though I never suggest to anyone that they might have experienced abuse, Andrea showed all the signs of a sexually abused woman: the way she walked, how she always looked down at the ground, holding her knees to her chest, and having a tendency to rock when she sat. Finally Andrea's mother, Phyllis, spoke, as she watched her daughter sway back and forth. "We want you to get better, Andrea. You don't deserve this life. You deserve to be a healthy young woman."

Andrea sneered at them. "You don't know what's happened to me. I don't deserve anything. I don't belong here; I belong out there. I know you don't want to hear that, though. I'm sorry I'm not the daughter you wanted."

I could see Andrea's mother flinch.

I joined in. "Now, Phyllis, why did you just do that?"

She looked at me blankly, shaking her head.

"You just flinched. What was it that Andrea just said that affected you?"

Phyllis looked down into the palms of her hands. "I guess . . . Oh." She stopped, debating whether to continue. "I've never told anybody this. It's just that before Andrea was born, I had prayed for a son. It wasn't that I didn't want a little girl. . . ."

I looked over to where Andrea now watched, fully engaged.

"What happened?" I asked, knowing how hard it is for parents to tell the secrets they have tried to protect their children from.

Phyllis looked down as she spoke, unable to meet anyone's eyes. "When I was little, I was molested by a neighbor boy. I thought that if I had a son, he wouldn't go through that. It was something that only happened to little girls, and so I didn't want a daughter; I didn't want her to experience the shame I felt."

Though Phyllis thought she was keeping her daughter safe by always imposing strict rules and harsh criticism upon Andrea, what she was really doing was repeating the cycle of abuse, demeaning Andrea's own experience as a child. Though Phyllis wasn't responsible for Andrea's addiction, she had, quite unwittingly, passed along her own unresolved shame.

Andrea shared later that she had always felt like damaged goods, but she didn't know why, and when her mother finally told her what happened, it was like a great weight was lifted. Andrea saw her mother as human for the first time that day, and upon empathizing with her mother's pain, Andrea walked over to Phyllis and offered her a Kleenex, taking her in her arms. Andrea told us later:

> I had so much shame I couldn't even say the word. Every time I talked, I was paralyzed with self-doubt and this idea that I didn't have anything worth sharing. I am still working on all of that—the fear and the shame, the self-doubt—but those are the times when I need to be gentle with myself, realizing that I am doing all of this for the first time. I see people going through this stuff, and I just want to tell them, "Hang on. Hang on. It gets better."

When a client is able to see where that shame comes from, we work through the trauma in two stages. He first voices whatever has happened to him from the child's point of view. He allows that most intimate self to come out and speak on his behalf. Then, after moving through the inner-child work, he brings his adult on board, becoming that child's advocate. Often folks in this situation were raised in a household where no one stuck up for them. Recovery grants them the opportunity to honor that space where they can feel the feelings, as Andrea did for her mother, offering their inner child the love, nurturance, respect, and attentiveness he or she was denied.

If you have been the victim of trauma or abuse, please get help now. There are many wonderful therapists and specialists working in this field who can begin to take you through the process of healing. This is precise work that needs to occur with the safety and supervision of a professional. If you were sick with a serious illness, you would find the right doctor, the means to pay, and the time in your schedule to treat it. Posttraumatic stress disorders are no different, requiring that you offer them the same reverence and commitment you would to the most critical of diseases.

WORKING THROUGH SHAME

Even if you have not experienced significant abuse, be gentle with yourself as you look back upon your life map.

Taking another colored pen, look through your life map to where you have suffered shame. Where in your story was there physical abuse? Sexual? Emotional? Intellectual? Spiritual? Did you learn in your childhood that you were of lesser value than your peers? Was this a message from your parents? Your siblings? Teachers? Preachers? Other adults?

As you look through your story, where did you carry shame? Did you feel bad for things that had occurred in your family or your life? Even things that had little or nothing to do with you? Did you feel that your family or school or church taught you a message that somehow you were a flawed human being? What did this message say? How was it emphasized or repeated throughout your history?

Our perpetrators should have carried their own shame, and as you move through this work, feel free to give it back to them. Go into a quiet, safe room and tell that person—your parent or that adult who passed along their shame unfairly—"I give you back your shame. I am not going to carry it anymore."

Yell it if you want to. Give it back! It is no longer yours to carry.

Guilt

I looked over to where Marlene sat slouched down on the ground after just trying to hurl the beanbag we use for anger exercises against the wall. At the age of fifty-eight, Marlene had been happily married for almost forty years, and had worked as a nurse for nearly as long, still committed to and impassioned about her job. For the last ten years, her ailing father had been living in Marlene's home, with Marlene as his main caretaker. Her brothers had not helped, and her mother passed away long ago.

Marlene looked down at a small stain on the carpet, an otherwise polite and charming woman who had just blown like a powder keg.

"What are you thinking about, Marlene?" I asked, watching her.

"I'm thinking you need to get this carpet steam-cleaned." She laughed.

"What's behind the joke?"

She stopped smiling, pausing as the group waited for her response, and then she began. "I'm thinking about how the person I am most angry at is me. I feel like I have treated my father like some great cross to bear. I don't even feel like I love him; he's just a patient, and I'm tired of taking care of him."

Before, Marlene had been beating the bag with our padded bat when suddenly the rage just came over her; she threw down the bat and lifted the bag into the air until we stopped her, coaxing her back down. Her anger had quickly morphed into pain, sadness sweeping over her, but there was still something missing, some key to the anger that she had yet to find.

"It's okay to be tired, to be frustrated, but that's not why you're so angry," I offered. "If it's you you're angry at, what did you ever do, Marlene? What moment brought that on?"

"I just feel so guilty," she shared. "I think about . . . oh, God, I think if only he passed away, I would be free. I wouldn't have to be a nurse at home and at work. He was always such a good father, so loving and protective of me, always watching out because I was the only girl. How could I wish for him to die?" Marlene choked out the words, her sobs taking over.

"Marlene, do you know that when my mother was dying, I would go visit her at the assisted living facility, and every time I would leave, I would hope that was the last time I was going to see her. And I loved my mother. I loved her so much I used to think I wouldn't be able to live without her. But, honey, it's not pretty watching anyone die, watching them suffer, and it's even harder when you're the one responsible for their welfare."

Like many caretakers, Marlene was bound to her patient and hated him for it. She thought this made her a bad person instead of realizing it just made her human. For years she had judged herself for her thoughts, believing she was supposed to be the perfect daughter, when what she was really doing was taking on the responsibility of her father's care, one that didn't need to be hers. And she began to eat because of it.

She would get angry with her father, leave the house, and then feel bad about her behavior. The guilt would consume her, and the food would assuage the guilt, allowing her, for a moment, to feel better. But then she would feel guilty about the food, and the cycle would continue. The guilt over her behavior would be trumped by her guilt over the food. The food would become the focus so she didn't have to look at herself.

When we don't know or understand that our guilt is natural, we think that feeling *bad* means we have done something *wrong*. In truth, we may have done nothing wrong. That feeling is instead a sign that we don't quite understand our value system around a certain behavior or thought. We need to check in with ourselves and see how we can alter the behavior or the value system to fit our lifestyle. We all do and say things we might deem horrible one day, but on another, we can see our words and actions in a new light, recognizing them as natural responses to stress and fear. When we trap ourselves in that guilt, we become immobilized, paralyzed in our behaviors. We believe that we must stick by our ineffective choices because we deserve what we have done.

Marlene was punishing herself for her thoughts by continuing to take care of her father. The situation wasn't healthy for anyone involved, most of all the elderly man who was at the resentful hands of a tired and burdened daughter. After that day when Marlene finally broke down, saying the truths she had been torturing herself with for a decade, she recognized that by continuing to take on the full responsibility of her father's care, she was creating a scenario that didn't fit her value system (which included treating her father with dignity and respect) and that she couldn't continue doing without causing further harm.

As Marlene prepared to leave, she shared with the group, "I found out that one of the most amazing things about guilt was that it kept me quiet. My thoughts were not that bad. They had just gotten worse in the silence of my brain."

UNCOVERING GUILT

Shame tells us we are a mistake, and guilt says we made one. For food addicts, we don't know how to handle mistakes, believing that they speak to our most intimate worth rather than our humanity. The feeling does not always mean we have done something wrong, but rather that we need to reassess our value systems and renegotiate our behaviors around them.

As you look through your life map, highlight, with the marker or pen you have chosen for guilt, the parts that you have never told anyone about. If there is something you initially left out of your life story, now is a good time to fill it back in. What are the things you have done or thought you did that you still feel guilty over? What are your secrets?

Looking back, how did food fit into this guilt cycle? Did you use food to suppress those feelings? Did you feel guilty for how you were using food? Do you see how guilt sets off the cycle of addiction when you overeat, or restrict, or binge and purge? Where did you feel immobilized, incapable of change or of taking action? When have you used denial to mask your feelings? When has guilt gotten between you and your relations? How has it affected those you love, and when have you carried it for others?

What has been your value system throughout your life? Can you identify it in your behaviors, able to see where you have followed it and where you have not?

Joy

For many people, joy describes everything that is great and beautiful and natural about our world and our lives, the ultimate expression of the loving, divine self. Through it come hope, healing, and spirituality, offering us the gifts of a healthy and honest life. But for so many, joy is worn like a mask, covering up all the emotions that one refuses to feel, convinced that as long as he or she is smiling, no one will know what's really going on.

I met Greg several years ago when he came to interview for a staff job at Shades. A counselor himself, he seemed hot-wired with joy, smiling, shaking hands, trying to impress. But I felt the whole show was not to get the job, but rather so we wouldn't notice what was obvious to anyone who shook Greg's small, bony hand. At that time, he had been suffering from anorexia for seven years, and though one would think that applying to be a counselor at an eating-disorder clinic would be ludicrous, such is the nature of denial. I told him as much at that time, explaining that we couldn't hire someone who might very well qualify as a client. He nodded and smiled and thanked me for my time.

Three years later he came back, weighing less than eighty pounds and finally ready to acknowledge that he needed help before he could continue offering it. Anorexics are incredibly tricky, because their high doesn't come from food; it comes from their own body chemicals. They play a dangerous game of chicken with their physical system, challenging it to starve so they can get high off the chemicals released when food is withheld. Because of this starvation—physically and mentally they are so depleted they are often unaware of what they are doing or how they can begin the work to heal. They have the highest fatality rate of any eating disorder, and we have tragically watched as some have passed through our doors never to recover.

But Greg was different. When he finally came into Shades, he could barely put a sentence together because of the significant malnutrition. But after nearly a year of working intensely on his recovery, we were able to get him up to a normal weight. We moved him into one of our halfway houses as he began his transition back into a normal life. After being denied the job at Shades years before, Greg began counseling troubled teens, and was looking forward to getting back to the job he loved so much. But as we approached his release date, Greg's weight began to rapidly drop, causing concern for our staff and his family. We put him back in a wheelchair, trying to get him to exert as few calories as possible. Though he had been living in transitional living, we insisted that he return to our residential house, where we would be able to better track and monitor his eating habits and weight.

I went over to his apartment the night before he was to resume living at the main center, walking in on him as he did push-ups in the living room. He stood up, nervous and ashamed, knowing that he was not supposed to be exercising at such a low weight. He practically jumped into his wheelchair, acting as though nothing had happened, smiling at me as though he had been awaiting my visit.

"Hi, Tennie, how was your day?"

"Mine was good, but I'm not here to talk about mine."

"Oh, no?"

"No. What were you doing?"

He faltered, looking around the room for an answer. "Nothing, I dropped something on the floor and was just looking for it."

"Hmm. What's going on, Greg?"

"What do you mean? I'm fine."

"You're in a wheelchair; I wouldn't call that fine. You are risking your life by trying to do those push-ups; you know that, don't you?"

He smiled even more, laughing. "Tennie, really I'm fine. I'm confused, too, about why I'm losing the weight, but I think it's just being out there, handing out applications, the job interviews. Really, I'm okay."

"There's a difference between okay and well, Greg. You are not well. You are a very sick man right now."

"Come on, you know I'll get the weight up," he cajoled. "I guess I just really like being here."

As much as Greg tried to convince everyone of his good cheer, the disguise was murdering him. His teeth jutted out of his skeletal face; the deep recesses of his eyes contradicted his smile as I fought my own tears at his image. Wishing I could find a way to get through to him, I asked, "Honey, have you ever actually experienced joy?"

"What? All the time."

"No, Greg, not when you force yourself to be happy so that everyone around you won't see your disease. That's not joy; that's a lie. Joy is believing in yourself, knowing that the world is here to love you and light your way. When have you felt that?"

The smile faded as Greg replied, "It's been awhile."

"When?"

He thought about it, recalling, "It was a few years ago. I was working with a client around Christmas. He had no family, you know. I mean, my life might have been tough, but I have a mom and dad. This kid didn't have anyone, and so I decided that on Christmas day, I would invite him to my family's house, and he was so happy, so filled with joy, that I saw my family in a new light. I saw how kind and generous my mother was, and though my dad doesn't say much, how he offered the boy the first slice of prime rib, reaching out to him in the only way he knew how. It was like my life had been muted and in black and white, and suddenly someone switched on the light. I never thought I could experience joy, and then, out of nowhere, it felt like that was possible for me. That's why I wanted to come here; I wanted to find that again." Greg looked down at his hands, the knuckles poking out of his skin. "I'm really thin, aren't I?"

"You are; it's why you're here. We want you to find that joy, Greg. It's what makes life worth living."

For so many eating-disorder folks, they are just filled with this false positivity. They run around like Pollyanna Positives, pretending the sun is always shining even when it's raining like hell out there. They are hysterical with joy—patting people, hugging them, offering everyone coffee and tea and cookies. You can barely get them to sit down, but beneath all that hysteria and happiness, they are the crying clowns.

They fear the idea of letting down that false front, exposing themselves to everyone, convinced that they will just drop off and hit rock bottom. Using all their energy to create that hysteria, they think they can't survive without it, and they leave no room in their reservoir for true and honest joy. I spent my whole life trying to make everyone around me happy and, in the process, made them miserable. I remember one of my first mentors, Anne, telling me that I was self-centered, and I replied, "What do you mean? I do everything for everyone. I work so hard for them. I just want them to be happy."

She replied, "Do you hear yourself? All you keep saying is, 'I, I, I.' Is that not self-centered?"

I had to realize that my false joy wasn't about other people; it was about me. I didn't have enough faith that God was going to take care of us, believing that it all came down to what I did. I thought that I had to be happy on the outside for the sake of my children, my husband, keeping that smile attached even when RL would get drunk and embarrass me in front of friends. I acted as if there was nothing wrong when my daughter Kim began to have trouble in school. I tried to float through on the surface, which meant I never got to touch down. I avoided all the real emotions that lead us to true joy, including pain, shame, guilt, and the rest. I relied on some decoy personality that I erroneously believed would protect me from the worst parts of myself. Anne was right—in my Pollyanna Positive mentality, I had become selfish and self-centered.

But then I began to pray, I began to meditate, and for once I could hear something more than just me. After Greg's return to our six-week residential program, his weight began to increase again, to the point where he was finally able to return to his profession, living close to the center so that we could continue to monitor his progress, the way any hospital might watch a cancer patient in miraculous remission . . . because Greg's recovery was nothing short of miraculous. He had finally begun to have active and conscious contact with his higher power, experiencing for the first time how prayer and meditation could help him to turn over the control that fueled his disease. He stopped by my office one after-

noon and told me, "In learning about meditation—the honor of silence—
I've learned how to create a relationship with God, and I've been better
able to see God's presence in my life and the lives of others. I believe that
all of us are called to do something. Our mission field is all around us. If
we do one thing to the best of our ability, then one person can touch one
person can touch one person. That is joy to me today."

DISCOVERING JOY

As we come to see and understand what real joy looks like, we are also
better able to recognize that divine self within, the ultimate manifestation of joy. Instead of grinning and bearing it, living our lives behind the
mask of "I'm fine, I'm fine, I'm fine" when really we are falling apart inside, we are able to experience life on life's terms as the person we were
always meant to be.

Pick up your last colored pen. Take a look at your life map and find
where you have worn that false mask of joy. When did you force yourself
to act happy? When have you forced others to do so? How have you used
the fronts of lookism and Pollyanna Positive to hide troublesome problems or issues in your life? Was your childhood infused with this false
sense that everything must look good? Everyone must act happy? When
has that attitude led you to hysteria, alienating you from your family,
friends, and peers?

Can you see when this behavior began? Were there times in your life
when the mask cracked? Did you break down, hit bottom, because you
just couldn't fake it anymore? Have you carried that joy for others?

I know one of the greatest reliefs in my life was when I finally stopped
smiling and instead learned how to laugh. I had spent my whole life
painting on that facade, and suddenly I didn't need to do that anymore.
I could cry when I needed to. I could use my voice. I learned to stand up

for myself in a true and powerful way, giving back my pain and shame and anger and guilt. Today I still attend many twelve-step meetings with people who understand. And I am now present to their stories, just as I can speak my own truths, laughing at the insane and painful things we have done. I no longer need to be a Pollyanna Positive; I am able to be me.

PART FIVE

Results

[A]nyone who stands on the edge of the unknown, fully in the present without reference point, experiences groundlessness. That's when our understanding goes deeper, when we find that the present moment is a pretty vulnerable place and that this can be completely unnerving and completely tender at the same time.

—Pema Chödrön

TEN

Healing Family

Bill's wife, Angie, sat across from me, distant if not a little hostile.

"Do you understand what I'm saying, Angie?" I questioned her, wondering whether she had been paying attention at all. Bill had just completed our six-day intensive program, but after we suggested he continue in our residential program for overeating, he replied that we would first have to explain the situation to his wife.

Angie knew about recovery, since she and Bill were both sober alcoholics. Years prior, they had entered Alcoholics Anonymous for their drinking, but Bill's overeating was a different story in her eyes.

Angie cleared her throat. "I guess what you're trying to tell me is that Bill's addiction to food is just like his alcoholism."

"In some ways, yes."

"Well, then, why can't he just continue in AA? Don't the steps there apply to his eating? Look at him; is he really that bad?"

Though Bill was only about eighty pounds overweight, our concern was *why* he was eating, using the food just as he did the alcohol as a means to suppress and control his emotions.

One of the biggest challenges for families is that so few people really understand what an eating disorder is. They immediately picture the most obese person or the most emaciated, unable to see that their child or their spouse might be the person with the disorder. If admitting to food addiction is difficult for the person with it, imagine how hard it can be for the families involved.

As Angie began to refocus on her nails, trying to ignore the conversation at hand, I interrupted, asking, "Do you want your husband to die?"

She looked up at me, taken aback, as I continued. "Eating disorders are a tricky, disturbing affliction, and just like any addiction, left untreated they will absolutely take the addict's life. In the case of your husband, it could be through heart disease, diabetes, stroke, heart attack. Whether it is the person who can't stop drinking or the person who can't stop eating, addiction is addiction is addiction."

"I get that. . . . I just don't understand why he has to go away to treat it," Angie argued. "He's needed at home—his children, his mother lives with us; his family comes first."

"What about his health? Angie, is this really about Bill? What was this week like for you?"

"What do you mean?"

"Did you all get on without him? Or did the whole place come tumbling down?"

She stopped, her face tightening, as I explained. "Wherever there's addiction, you're bound to find some codependency. Sounds like you've got a bit going on there. Because though our families do come first, how can we be there for our families when we can't be there for ourselves?"

For families of addicts, they aren't sure whether they would die without the addict or whether they want to kill him or her. But they do think that if only they could control them, the outcome might look better. For Angie, she had been using recovery to deny Bill's addiction to food, believing that just because he was in AA, that meant he didn't need anything else, that his solution could be found at home. But Bill's addiction went beyond alcohol; it even went beyond food, straight into the heart of the codependency that neither Angie nor Bill wanted to face. But as they both soon learned, everything in recovery has to be renegotiated.

Setting Boundaries

Most addicts use their dependency as a buffer between them and their relationships, which is why the world can be a scary place when they finally surrender addiction. After they take the substance out, they must redefine those relationships, learning to set boundaries with their family, friends, and even coworkers. I know people who have been abstinent a couple of years who can do the family dinner and manage the fight about who was supposed to bring the turkey and who was supposed to bring the ham. They're able to see it all in realistic perspective, and not be overwhelmed by the personalities involved. But early on in their recovery, food addicts are so raw, they don't know how to handle those confrontations. They can be triggered by the stress of the family dynamic, falling back on their addictions in order to cope. Boundaries help us to navigate that dynamic, help us begin to assert what we can and cannot handle, and whom we can and cannot trust.

Pull out those letters to your parents you wrote in part two, and take a look at how those messages have affected all your relationships. Throughout this chapter, use the letters to identify how your parents taught you either to set or to ignore boundaries in your life. How did they influence your self-concept? How have you made decisions in your life or created behaviors around those boundaries? How have their messages affected how you view your body, how you process emotions, and how you create intimacy?

As Pia Mellody explains, "Codependents demonstrate the boundary systems that their parents had. If the parents' boundaries were nonexistent, the children usually do not develop any boundaries either. If the parents had damaged boundaries, the children almost always develop boundary systems damaged in the same way."

In shaping new boundaries, we transform the family dynamic in which we were raised into a new system, with renegotiated rules, relationships, and beliefs, and a healthier perspective on how to receive and give those messages that are the basis of development.

For Bill, it was hard enough to admit he had a problem and to ask for help, but to hear his wife push back, demeaning his weight gain and his addiction, he lost whatever initial conviction he might have had.

I walked him back to the car after Angie left to use the ladies' room. They were returning home after Bill had decided that he wouldn't stay.

"I just think they really need me," he explained halfheartedly.

"Bill, *need* is just another word for codependency. Being with families is one of the most important things in our lives, but if you can't put your life on hold for six weeks in order to get healthy, then where do you fall on that priority list?"

Bill began to rub his neck, hoping he could just get out of Dodge as I continued. "My whole life I walked on eggshells around the alcoholics I knew, and my children walked on eggshells around me. Addiction wasn't innocuous; it came out in all sorts of forms: my anger, my inability to pay attention, the fact that I was always thinking about what I was going to eat or do next. I could never be present to the people I loved. Even when I was so far up their butts, telling them what to do or trying to be a good parent, I could never just relax, because that need for food was always driving me."

Bill laughed as he said, "I used to think when God made me, He forgot to add the food."

"I know—me, too. It completed me, but that meant there wasn't a whole lot of room for my loved ones."

For some families, the addiction concept is easy to swallow; for others, it can be incredibly difficult. The family doesn't understand why some people can eat normally and others can't. They think it is a question of willpower, not understanding that when an addict's pain exceeds his or her willpower, that addict is going to use.

Angie walked up, and she could see from the look in Bill's eyes that he was staying.

"I don't know how you think you can do this," she began to yell, nearly shrieking at him in the parking lot. "You have responsibilities; you have people to take care of. . . ."

Bill put his hands softly but firmly on her shoulders, facing her. She stopped, confused as to what he was doing. "When you yell at me," he began, "I think you don't love or respect me, and I feel shame and fear and pain. I need you to understand why I am doing this. I intend to be there for you, but I also need to be there for me."

Angie stared at him, dumbstruck. Finally she responded, "I respect you, Bill. I love you."

He smiled. "Then I need you to respect my decision."

BUILDING CONFRONTATIONS

Confrontations are a way to call to someone's attention how that person's behavior is affecting us, and setting the boundaries for how we would like to be treated. When we confront someone, we are sharing our feelings (choosing from one of the seven basic emotions to keep things simple), while at the same time suggesting a different action we would want that other person to take. We then offer how we might also do things differently, showing what we need to do for ourselves and the other person in order to process that feeling. These confrontations, as Bill so powerfully demonstrated, give us the language by which to create our boundaries. We are able to communicate to others what we can and cannot withstand, and offer solutions to problems we might otherwise sweep under the rug, ignoring them until they become resentments.

A typical confrontation looks like this:

When you do:
I think:
I feel:
I need/would like:
I intend to:

Think about whom in your life you need to confront and how you would deliver that message, respecting their needs and boundaries while still communicating your own. Perhaps start with the top five people (parents, siblings, spouse, children, coworkers, etc.) who you feel need to better respect your boundaries. As we move through this chapter, you will have a better idea of who those folks might be, and how they should be addressed. Practice your confrontations in the mirror, getting used to this new language. This is a learning experience. You might not be that comfortable with the confrontations at first, stammering through as you try to set those early fragile boundaries, but over time, you will see how they can help to renegotiate your life in recovery.

Be prepared for all types of reactions, knowing that confrontations are supposed to be hard. Not everyone will accept your confrontations with the grace and compassion that Angie exhibited. But if you take the risk, you will find out more about your relationships than you ever knew was possible.

THE FIRST WALL

External systems are all about the body and what we look like. When we set external boundaries, we protect our body and control the space between ourselves and other people, creating our first wall of defense against the world. Everybody has the right to their own physical space, but when someone violates our space, they disrespect our boundaries. And often we are the ones who give them unintended permission to do this.

By the end of Cheryl's first day, she was best friends with all of Shades—offering them tissues and making sure that everyone had a pillow when they sat down. Cheryl was a sweet-talking African American woman from Alabama who weighed close to four hundred pounds. With her hot-pink sweats and big hoop earrings, she had enough personality for the whole town. By the second day, I walked in on her hugging the daylights out of another client, who seemed uncomfortable with Cheryl's onslaught of affection. The client was an anorexic who probably hadn't been touched in a decade, and there Cheryl was like some overgrown retriever, knocking the poor woman down.

"Cheryl, I want you to let go of that woman right now," I interrupted.

She did so immediately, scared by my tone as I continued. "I don't want you touching anyone else while you're here."

"But she was sad," Cheryl began.

"Good, she needs to feel sad. She's been starving that feeling away, and she doesn't need you to interrupt her process. When we let people in, it should be because we want them to come in and have given them permission to do so. You can't just go up and take over someone else's space. You cannot kiss or touch or even hug someone without their permission."

For so many, this is a lot harder than it should be. I know that growing up, I was the exact opposite of Cheryl but for the same reason: I shunned the very attention I craved. I wanted to be hugged, but I hated to be touched. My physical boundaries were so screwed up, it wasn't until I could begin to have healthy boundaries in that area that I became more comfortable with giving and receiving embraces.

I shared this with Cheryl as the crocodile tears began to form in her eyes. "Now, honey, I love hugging people; I get it. Hugging is a very important form of affection. We do it all the time. But we need to allow others to tell us how they want to be touched. Once we know how to touch them, we'll know how to treat them."

Cheryl fought back her tears. "No one ever hugged me growing up."

"I know. No one ever hugged me either, but that's why we learn to build boundaries, respecting others so that they can respect ours. That way we all learn how to touch and hug, receiving the love that should have always been ours."

The simple question, "May I give you a hug?" can absolutely change how someone feels. You are offering the comfort of affection while still respecting that person's space and ability to receive it.

Setting boundaries is not about erasing the connection between you and your loved ones. Once we are able to reject that "all or nothing" mentality, reducing the polarization that addiction creates, boundaries can be loosened and tightened in any relationship. Though at first the pendulum might swing all the way to one side and then all the way back the other direction, we have to keep working until the pendulum finds itself in the middle. There, we will strike a balance between respecting our relationships and respecting ourselves.

Take a look at those letters you wrote to your parents, and identify how you developed your external systems. Look at the messages you received about your body. How was the body regarded in your house? Was it respected? Was yours respected? What did you learn about physical intimacy? How do you see those messages reflected in your present relationships? Is there a confrontation that needs to be made in your life today in order to rebuild your physical boundaries? Begin to observe how you offer affection to others and how you respond to it. What kind of boundaries do you need to build in order to protect your body today?

CREATING EMOTIONAL BALANCE

When we set up internal boundaries, we are protecting our thoughts, feelings, and behaviors. We are deciding how we are going to process incoming data, in the hopes of finding emotional balance. When someone is in addiction, it is like no one is home, but as the addict begins to clean up and get healthy, she begins to feel again. This is where she must protect that internal system, developing boundaries to manage those emotions.

When Nadia's mother, Elena, dropped her off at Shades, waiting to speak with me before she could leave her thirty-four-year-old daughter in our care, I knew Nadia was going to have an interesting path before her.

Elena stood to greet me when I walked in, telling me that Nadia had been an overeater since she was five. "It was something I always tried to control, you know," she explained. "I saw it; I knew it was a problem, but everyone would tell me she was just a little girl. Little girls shouldn't be on diets. I know it sounds crazy, but I tried everything—Weight Watchers, Nutrisystem, I even hired her a personal trainer."

"When she was how old?"

"It started in elementary school, but it's lasted forever. I just wanted to tell you that I wouldn't be surprised or disappointed if this doesn't work. Nothing's worked."

"Elena, does Nadia still live with you?" I asked.

"Yes, of course. I help her with her diets."

"And she's still sixty pounds overweight?"

"Yes." Elena looked down like she had failed, disappointed in herself.

"That's not your fault, Elena. Food addiction can't be healed by any-one but the addict. It's up to Nadia to want to change, to stop using her food to manipulate and control her environment. It sounds like you've dedicated much of your life to her eating habits, and yet still both of you are miserable."

Nadia was an overeater who had spent her last few years living at home, sleeping in her childhood bedroom, though she was approaching thirty-five. Elena did everything for her—shopping for her, styling her hair, treating her like a little doll, and, as I saw when she returned for Family Week, speaking for her grown daughter.

After Nadia got to Shades, she started making friends, coming out of the shell in which she lived, beginning to laugh with peers and enjoy herself. But once Elena joined us for Family Week, Nadia went back to acting like the sick and depressed woman who had arrived three weeks before.

"How are you feeling?" I asked Nadia one morning at breakfast as she shoved some breakfast ham to the other side of her plate, ignoring me. "I just asked you a question, Nadia," I tried again, but Elena jumped in before she had a chance to respond.

"She's fine, just a little tired, I think. It's been a long week," she ex-plained, referring to Family Week.

"I was talking to your daughter," I replied. "But I guess then I should ask you, how are you doing?"

"Oh, it's hard. I mean, I've been struggling for so many years. She's always like this." Elena began to rub her daughter's back.

"She wasn't last week. Nadia, tell me what happened to the girl I met before Family Week started, the one who had the whole table laughing at breakfast, the one who often would be the first to speak, to share. Where did she go?"

Nadia just shrugged. Later, I stopped by Nadia's room, catching her as she lay in her bed, writing in her journal.

She looked up as I stood in her doorway. Putting down her pen, she quietly said, "I know you're disappointed in me."

"It doesn't really matter what I think. Are you disappointed in you?"

"I guess I just feel like that's what my mom expects from me. She feels good when I feel bad. Does that make any sense?"

I sat down. "Absolutely—it's called enmeshment, but you don't have to be sick just because your mother's here. You have the real possibility for change, Nadia. You're getting treatment, and from what I saw last week, you want to be alive. You want friends and a normal shot at this existence. But what you have to realize is that your mother might never change. She is also an unhealthy woman. She is bound to her codependency, and unless she is willing to do the work, she will end up being sicker than you."

It was Nadia who had to change. She had allowed her feelings and behaviors to be dictated by what Elena thought they should be. Lost in the codependency, she didn't know how to feel, looking to her mother for all her cues. In order to maintain her recovery around her mother, Nadia had to renegotiate her boundaries.

By the fourth day of Family Week, Elena watched as her daughter returned to being that light and engaging spirit she had been for her first few weeks. She didn't know what to do, ultimately breaking down crying in one of our group sessions. Elena was confused as to why Nadia was able to heal at Shades and not at home. When someone is addicted, the whole family is engaged in addiction, and it can be just as challenging for the family to surrender their behaviors as it is for the addict.

This is why it is so important to engage our families in recovery, because if they aren't brought along in the process, they will sabotage the addict's progress.

Take a moment to visualize what your internal boundaries look like. Are they like walls that no one can traverse, or are they perforated, showing where they have been damaged before? Are you strong in some areas and fearful in others? Do you have no boundaries whatsoever? Are people easily able to attack you, or do you have healthy boundaries so that you are able to filter what people say to you without shutting down completely? In order to begin strengthening the internal system, you must be willing to take control of what information you allow in.

For many, this is a whole new way of thinking. You are not responsible for other people's actions or behaviors, but you are responsible for yours. You are the architect of your thoughts and the director of your feelings. This doesn't mean that you don't engage in relationships with other people or that you don't respond to them emotionally, but you are in control of what that response might be. If harm is done, you do not need to carry the burden. If you caused it, you can make amends. Our goal is to create a personal shield that protects us from the flaming arrows of other people's words, stopping them before they get to our hearts, and yet still allowing the emotions to enter. That sounds like a herculean task, but, really, it isn't.

If you hear a message that is going to trigger that addictive response, the anxiety that negativity engenders, you need to be able to say, "Hmm, that's interesting, but that's not what I think or what I feel, so I will set it aside and look at it later to see whether there is anything valid to be learned from it." Ask for God's help in being able to see that lesson, and then let those words go.

It takes six weeks to break an old habit and six weeks to start a new one. Our brains are wired to do what they know. They are like a computer that runs on whatever program it is being given, no matter what kind of bugs that program might have. But if you create a new program and try it out for an extended period of time, your brain will start running on that course. Take pause at every opportunity you have, and remove yourself from the comment or behavior that is piercing your armor, and it should take only six weeks to change that unhealthy process of boundary breaking.

Does this mean we are always able to keep our internal boundaries up all the time? We would hardly be human if we could. We are going to get our feelings hurt, becoming upset when someone doesn't treat us the way we'd like or when things don't go our way. But if we are able to keep our internal boundaries in mind, we will be better able to control our reactions.

Reviewing the letters to your parents, where were your internal boundaries crossed with them and where are they crossed today? Where could you have been stronger with others and where could you have let them in more? Where have you allowed family and friends to influence your thoughts and feelings and when have you been the major offender? How have you offended?

Looking forward, what steps can you take to create healthy boundaries with your parents? Your siblings? Your spouse? Your children? Does a confrontation need to be made to create or mend your emotional boundaries? By securing these boundaries with those you love most, you will be able to secure them everywhere in your life.

Good Orderly Direction

When I first came into recovery, I was taught that GOD stands for *good orderly direction*. In order to have GOD in our lives, we have to build boundaries to protect our spiritual systems. Those systems make up our moral fiber, defining how we choose to be intimate with others. In establishing our spiritual boundaries, we shape our sexual ones. This is not a matter of shame or judgment, but rather choosing a value system that works for you and then staying true to those values.

From sixty-year-old virgins to sixty-year-old prostitutes, I have seen it all, but the one thing all these clients share is that their most intimate choices are often based on how they perceive their value. Every person has the right to be sexual with whomever he or she wants in whatever manner he or she chooses; anything outside of that is breaking a boundary, or even the law. If someone is coercing you into a behavior or act, you are giving away a piece of your soul that will be very difficult to get back. Anytime we do something we don't want to do, we are relinquishing a part of ourselves.

Codependency is like a diamond with countless facets. On the one hand, addicts feel that they don't possess enough worth and always need someone to take care of them. Needing people to fill that hole in the soul, they get lost in others and often have trouble separating themselves from them. Antidependents, however, would rather have no one involved in their lives. We see this a lot in anorexics who get so isolated from other humans that they want no contact at all, becoming spiritually and sexually anorexic. Either way, codependency and antidependency are both born from unhealthy boundaries with other people, and are often the source of unhealthy relationships.

It was Tracy's last week at Shades when she finally cracked, allowing us into the horrific world of sex slavery in which she had lived the majority of her adult life. A thirty-year-old woman with golden brown eyes and jet-black hair, she had a striking presence. After being saved by a Christian organization, she came to the United States from the Philippines, determined to set out on a new life, but found herself mired in depression. She started starving herself, though she couldn't understand why. For so many years, she dreamed of being able to eat.

The same organization that helped her before came to her aid again when one of its representatives went to visit Tracy, only to discover she weighed less than seventy pounds and was living in squalor. For the first five weeks of her stay, she kept to herself. Adamant that the language barrier was too much to overcome, she refrained from saying anything more than she had to. She knew that her sponsor from the organization would be checking in on her progress once she was released, and so, in a last-ditch effort, she sat down to write out her life story. She didn't get very far before she hurled the workbook across the room and raced out of the building. She ran into the road and in front of an oncoming car, indifferent to whether it hit her. Fortunately, it didn't.

One of our staff was able to calm her down, bringing her back into the living room, where most of our clients spend their time relaxing and socializing when they are not working on their recovery. My daughter Karen made it there first as Tracy finally shared the terrible tale of her childhood. She cried as she told Karen that she didn't believe recovery would work for her. I joined Karen not long after, sitting down next to Tracy. She flinched from my presence.

"Am I sitting too close?" I asked.

"I don't like to be touched."

"I'm sure you don't—you've had enough people in your life disrespect your boundaries."

She nodded, quiet as she practically melted into the couch, her small frame camouflaged by the cushions.

"What made you get so upset, Tracy?"

She shrugged, looking at me blankly.

"I understand if you don't feel comfortable talking with me about your past. It's okay; you can tell whomever you want, but I'm just wondering: What were you working on that made you run out of here and nearly hurt yourself?"

She stared down at her hands. "The inventory asked about our sex lives now. One of the questions was whether I break my boundaries in my life today."

"All right, and why did that get you so upset?" Tracy's back straightened, her fear palpable. I continued. "Stay with that feeling; you're safe now, sweetheart. We only want to protect you."

"I still prostitute myself. I don't even need the money, but it's the only thing I know to do. I keep doing it and I hate myself, and I want to be different but nothing changes. It is who I am."

Tracy's sexual abuse as a child had influenced her entire spiritual system. Unable to see herself as a perfect child of God, she saw herself as a damaged, worthless person, incapable of receiving affection unless she was selling herself. Tracy had her rights taken from her time and time again, and when she came to us, her spiritual boundaries were impenetrable to anyone who wanted to help her.

If you treat the eating disorder, you will treat the codependency, so we started there. Tracy was with us for six months, and at first the work was slow going, but eventually she began to take direction, helping out around the meal hall, even laughing with others during the gym hour. When we suggested she begin working with a sponsor, she asked for someone with many years of abstinence who had also been sexually abused. She started taking good orderly direction from someone she could trust, and she began to rebuild those spiritual boundaries she had never had the chance to have.

Many addicts have such compromised spiritual systems due to their addictions that they are building them as though for the first time. Once they begin the work in recovery, they must identify what it means to be comfortable in intimacy. According to Robert Burney, author of *Codependence: The Dance of Wounded Souls,* "The simplest and most understandable way I have ever heard intimacy described is by breaking the word down: *into me see.* That is what intimacy is about—allowing another person to see into us, sharing who we are with another person." For so long the addict has been in relationship with the addiction, but now he gets to be in relationship with other people, either requiring him to see his current sexual partner (or partners) in a new light or recognizing that such partnership is possible.

As you look over your letters to your parents, how has your spiritual system been affected by the messages you were taught? How did your parents treat or reflect sexual intimacy in the household? Was there overt sexual abuse—were you touched or forced to do anything sexually? Or was there covert abuse—did you see sexual behaviors or materials that were not age-appropriate? Was sexuality discussed at all? What messages did you receive about it? Religious? Scientific? Moral? How do these messages get mirrored in your sexual boundaries today? How can you begin to create good orderly direction in response?

Looking forward, what kind of intimacy are you looking for today? What kind of partnership? Do you need to confront someone or even yourself in order to repair your spiritual and sexual boundaries? What would your ideal coupleship look like? Are you in that relationship right now? If not, what boundaries do you need to set in order to create "into me see" in your life?

Facing Codependency

When my mother was in her late seventies, I was presented with the choice many adult children face as their parents age: to keep her in my home despite her failing health, or to find an assisted-living facility that would be better suited to take care of her. Though assisted living would finally force her off of her drugs and booze, though I recognized that it would have been emotionally disastrous for her to live with me, though I had been taking care of her my whole life, I was absolutely torn up about it. I knew I needed to make the decision, and on a trip to Florida I decided to take a walk along the beach and consider my options.

In normal, healthy parenting, the energy relationship should be from the parent to the child. The parent gives care to the child, raising her with all the tools she needs to survive and thrive in the world. The parents offer that child an understanding of what a healthy relationship looks like so the child might seek out what she knows, finding herself in a healthy, sustainable relationship like the one exhibited by her parents.

Few of us, however, are actually raised in that scenario. Instead, we find ourselves dancing the dance of dysfunction, just as most of us watched our parents do. With an alcoholic husband, mother, and daughter, I was good at caring for others. I knew when to throw them in the shower, when to force them to drink charcoal, and when to call 911. It was my job, and I was proud that I could get it done without the neighbors knowing.

As I took that fateful walk on the beach, I reflected on what I had learned in recovery: that there are times when people need to take care of themselves. We have to let them go and know that they are protected by God's care rather than our control. For so long I had received esteem from playing my mother's mother, and finally, at the age of forty-two, I decided it might be time for me to relinquish my role. Having suffered the consequences of my mother's addiction all my life, swearing I would never be like her, I continued to enable the behaviors I so despised. And I knew that I didn't need to do that anymore. I stopped along my walk and looked out into the ocean, where I saw a small sailboat. All of a sudden I had this vision of my mother on that boat, in a little sailor's outfit with the hat and all, and she was waving at me, saying, "Tennie, I'll be all right. I'm fine."

Instead of continuing to take care of that woman, facilitating her alcoholism and drug addiction, I turned her care over to people I thought might do a better job. Just as we were able to work with Nadia in ways her mother never could, assisted living ended up being the best choice for my mother. She never drank again, living out her days among her peers, more independent than she had been her whole life.

We have all been enablers and we have all enabled, because addiction is a family disease. It forces us all into its dance, aiding and abetting even when we believe we are only trying to help. Think about who might be enabling in your life, or, if you are the only addict, think about who is your primary enabler. There are three simple questions to determine whether you are enabling or being enabled:

1. *Is it really helping?* In supporting the addict, are you helping them toward recovery or are you helping them in their addiction? Is the safety net being cast going to save them or you, or allow you both to fall even deeper?
2. *Whose responsibility is it?* Are you responsible for someone else's disease or should they begin taking accountability? If you are taking care of them, you are not helping; you are carrying the burden of their addiction. If someone is taking care of you, are you ready to take that responsibility back?
3. *What are your motives?* Why are you helping and what do you receive from it? Are you protecting the addict, your family, yourself, and do you take pride in that protection?

As a family member or partner of someone struggling with addiction, I have learned that there is much you can do to help your loved one while still allowing him or her to take responsibility for his or her disease. I cannot say how many times I have said the serenity prayer in my life, and I try to practice its teaching on a daily basis. But when I was dealing with my mother's, my daughter's, and my husband's addictions, those words were my hotline to God:

God, grant me the serenity to accept the things I cannot change,
The courage to change the things I can,
And the wisdom to know the difference.

The scariest thing we can do is let go, but if we don't, we are participating in the suicide of our loved one. If you're an addict, you have an enabler, and you need to ask yourself, "Who is that person in my life?" You can stop accepting his or her help today. Instead, you can face the consequences and start accepting the things you cannot change.

If you are enabling someone, look at how you are doing so. Is it financial? Physical? Emotional? Spiritual? What are you giving him or her that he or she needs to find on their own? And what is it going to take for you to stop?

Break the Cycle Now

After Bill completed his treatment at Shades, he returned home to continue in Alcoholics Anonymous as well as Overeaters Anonymous, but problems began to arise between him and Angie. She didn't want to eat what was on his meal plan, and he found himself relapsing with food because he couldn't keep his boundaries with her. They were both dedicated to their own recoveries, but they became at odds in their relationship.

Though they had weathered alcoholism, overeating, recovery, and codependency, they had long forgotten why they had fallen in love. I know when I started to heal I felt the same way. I was prepared to leave RL, even though we were both in programs of recovery. Though both free from addiction, we had never gotten to know each other, only the addict.

On the day I planned to tell RL I was leaving, I walked through our front door and something in me finally broke. I saw him sitting there reading his newspaper, and I knew in that moment that he loved me; he just didn't know how to show it. Instead of announcing my departure, I went over to him and took the newspaper out of his hands. I crawled up onto his lap and I put my arms around him. As we both began to cry, we began a new journey toward love.

The irony of addiction is that a craving lasts only fifteen minutes. We wage war our whole lives against a battle that lasts a measly quarter of an hour. But if it were just the craving, just the piece of cake, only the call to the pizza joint that delivers in thirty minutes or less, we would just sit with the craving, allow it to pass, and be finished with it. But so much of how we think and feel and behave is caught up in how we relate to other people, and that takes longer than fifteen minutes. Those relationships form the root of addiction, building up over the years and demanding the space to heal.

Bill called me six months after he left treatment to tell me that he and Angie were separating.

"Hmmm," I replied. "How long have you been abstinent?"

"Six months," he said proudly.

"And how long has Angie been going to Co-Dependents Anonymous?"

"I guess the same time."

"You know that it's suggested that we don't make any major changes in our first year of recovery. It doesn't matter that you have both been sober; the same goes for your new recoveries."

"I know, Tennie," he responded. "But it just ain't working."

"Sometimes it's little by slow, Bill. We can't just change everything and think that it's going to be smooth sailing. You both have a family system that you have built and created over twenty years together, and it is going to take more than six months to make the necessary changes to that dynamic."

That family system is everything. It imposes its patterns on everyone involved, forcing them to mimic, migrate, and head back to what is familiar until it no longer works. And then the family reaches for a new set of patterns, a new way to live. This is what twelve-step recovery offers to all of us.

"What do you suggest, then?" Bill asked.

"I suggest you stay at the dance with the one you brought, and take a little bit more time to learn this new routine, loving each other into the same rhythm. It might not be easy right now, but you can have your money back if I ever told you that recovery was going to be easy."

Through abstinent living, we can create a new framework—not one that demands the world be perfect, but rather one that trusts that the world is turning just as it should. If we are willing to stand in the presence that intimacy requires, those pieces that at one time looked so separate, so incapable of healing come together. We curl up into each other's laps, having been given permission to give and receive the affection we have always wanted, and we begin that new journey into love.

ELEVEN

Feelings Embraced

*I*t was one of the last sessions of our six-day intensive program, and we were going around our circle, the clients discussing what their next steps were to be. Would they continue in a recovery program? Did they need to stay on at Shades? What life changes did they need to make at home and in their relationships? And finally, what would their meal plan look like? Margaret stared at the after-care plan we had just given her, which suggested she continue on our meal plan, attend Overeaters Anonymous meetings, and abstain from sugar, white flour, and nicotine. Though everyone else was nearly giddy as they reviewed their sheets, clutching them like well-earned degrees, Margaret held hers in disdain, a dark pall washing over her face.

After the person next to Margaret shared his reaction, hopeful about what his future might bring, we reached Margaret, who glanced up at everyone and replied blankly, "I can't do this."

I watched her foot begin to shake, her anxiety and discomfort translated through it, wagging at all of us. "That's fair, Margaret. What are you feeling in this moment that makes you think you can't do it?"

She looked back down at the paper and her foot sped up. "I don't know."

"Yes, you do. You've known all along."

She looked back up at me. "Fear?"

"Is that a question or is that how you're feeling?"

She shook her head slowly, her foot breaking its tempo and then picking back up again. "I'm just afraid that if I can't do this and I fail, I'll have nothing left. I'll just be hopeless."

Fear is one of the biggest obstacles to change, telling us we're incapable, that to try to do something different is not only impossible but ludicrous. I asked her, "Do you see what you're doing with your foot?"

Margaret stopped it immediately and responded, "I'm not doing anything."

"You were. You were shaking that foot like you couldn't wait to get out of here, couldn't wait to have a cigarette, go to McDonald's, be through with this."

Margaret shrugged.

"Margaret, awareness is ninety-nine percent of any solution. I know you won't necessarily walk out of here and never have a cheeseburger, a cigarette, or a bowl of ice cream again. Hell, you might get that on the way home, but what you can start doing is being aware. Stop yourself as you're sitting at the drive-through or combing through your purse for a lighter, and recognize how you're feeling. See if you might be able to embrace it. Maybe just for that moment, you can take the opportunity not to smoke, not to order the french fries. Just for that moment."

Margaret had been battling her weight since she was six years old, smoking and eating herself to her first heart attack at fifty-four. Now fifty-seven, she knew that if she didn't start changing things soon, she was sure to be dead by seventy. She would miss out on watching her grandchildren grow, on being able to age with her husband. She was battling decades of bad habits, but that didn't make her any less capable than the rest of the group.

So much of our lives has been driven by fear—we are afraid of what we are not going to get, and once we get it, we are afraid of what we are going to lose. But when we offer ourselves the simple gift of awareness, we become present. Holding on to that moment of fear, the passing of pain, we change directions. We create new habits from the old, and find adventure in place of hunger.

Let's take a long, hard look at that life map from part four. Is it covered in all the different colors of your denied and carried feelings? Can you see how you have consistently covered up your true self, hiding from your adventure because you feared what it held? Where have you failed to set boundaries or broken ones previously set? Are you able to recognize when you ate instead of stopping in the moment and processing the emotion at hand? All of those colors represent food. They represent the substances and processes we have used to hide from the core issues of our lives. They have covered us up, at first like a warm blanket, but in the end, they only offer counterfeit comfort. After time, that blanket gets tighter, becoming a straitjacket, pinning us to behaviors that only hurt.

By the end of my addiction, I was absolutely disconnected from my present, unable to sit in anything. I, too, shook like a leaf whenever I was presented with something I didn't like. I remember those meetings Allen referred to when he first told me I was a bulimic. Someone would disagree with me, or challenge my opinion on a client, and I didn't know how to accept anything but my own will. I thought that if I worked hard enough, studied hard enough, spoke loudly enough, people would give me the right of way. They would allow me to control every decision in whatever landscape I was working—home, work, social engagements. I knew I was a bully, even if I was ignorant of the fact that I was a bulimic. But when someone would challenge me, or suggest I do or behave differently, my right leg would start quaking, kicking out in defiance and mistrust.

I could feel nothing but compassion for Margaret that morning, because I had once been where she sat, believing that I alone was going to have to solve my eating disorder, and knowing that if it were left to me, I had little to hope for. But Dr. Hollis had looked at me with the same empathy I share with my clients, explaining to me that I didn't have to worry about forever. And I didn't have to do it alone. All I had to do was trust in God for one moment, one moment at a time, and reach out to others whenever I got scared. It wasn't about willpower, about digging my feet in and fighting to the death; it was about surrendering to those feelings, allowing myself to relax in their embrace.

Each feeling offers us a powerful gift to aid us in this adventure. I remember when my grandchildren were little and they would play these video games where the main character would have to jump and hit certain items in order to complete various levels. Each time, the little guy in the video game would gain some treasure or gift upon his success, and I would laugh, thinking that in real life, I was just learning to play the same game. We called it recovery. And with it, I became ever watchful of the gifts that lay in my path, acquiring the skills needed for a healthy life. Yes, there were trials, setbacks, hard days and challenging moments, but as I overcame them I grew, gaining some treasure I did not even know was available to me. And which can now be available to you.

Embraced Self-Concept

Sylvia Plath once wrote, "I took a deep breath and listened to the old bray of my heart. I am. I am. I am." You are. You have always been. Underneath that dirty old blanket of your addiction lies a powerful man or woman just waiting to emerge: feelings processed, boundaries set, and with a new tape playing in that head. Look back over your initial self-concept, those letters to your parents, the body-image work and inner-child messaging. Review your life history and confrontations, and begin to see who that divine self really is. Pull out some paper or go to work in your journal and write a description of this new self-concept. This is the person who lives free of addiction, who is able to embrace his or her feelings, and who has the courage to develop healthy relationships. It should be a realistic mental image, with achievable goals and ideas about your future. Describe how you plan to change your behaviors (your goals around eating, smoking, shopping, drinking, spending, gambling). What new activities would you like to participate in (hobbies, jobs, volunteer work)? And what kind of new belief systems and boundaries do you need to create around your relationship with yourself, your family, friends, work associates, and the God of your understanding?

As we consider the gifts that can come from embracing your feelings, see how you can build upon that concept. Where does this new person embrace fear? How does she process anger? How does he express joy? Once this work is completed, you should read that description twice a week for six months. Get to know that person. See how he or she changes. How does she respond to life? How does he manage his food? Keep that person in mind as we move into the meal plan. You are no longer eating to hide that authentic divine self, but rather to nourish your new self-concept.

ENERGY

Probably one of the last feelings to really challenge me was rage. Even after I came home from treatment, I didn't know how to embrace my anger, convinced that the only way for people to hear me was to scream. I remember the last time this happened, almost fifteen years ago. We had hired an executive director at Shades, because I needed to take some time away from the director's position; I was exhausted by both running Shades of Hope and working as one of its counselors. I continued on as a therapist and as a partial owner. Though I had hired John to run the place, technically I was still his boss. One day I saw a big pile of rocks sitting in front of our main administrative building, leftovers from a recent landscaping project. I told John that they needed to be moved, concerned that a staff member or client could trip over them, to which he replied, "No problem. I'll take care of it."

The next day, I came back to the center and the rocks were still there. John apologized and said he would make a call right away, but by the third day, when I got to the center and the rocks hadn't moved, I lost my mind. I don't even remember the things I yelled at that poor man. That old rage just came over me, taking me out of the present and pushing me into behaviors I thought I had left behind. I made those rocks personal. Instead of realizing this was a busy man who had a lot to do and had simply overlooked a small task, I decided it was an insult to me. That those rocks were a sign of his disrespect. Going back into that child mind that sees everything from only our perspective, I fought back— personally attacking our director and his character.

There were people around—the clients and staff I had previously been so concerned about—but that didn't matter. After I was through with John, I went to the maintenance shed, grabbed a shovel, and started moving the rocks myself. My daughters, the staff, even my husband all tried to stop me, but I was unrelenting. I screamed at all of them as I carried the rocks down to a nearby creek bed.

It took me hours to see what I was doing. When new folks come into Shades, they often do so dragging a heavy weight, a boulder of drama and unprocessed emotions, that bag of old dead chickens, and we tell them that in order to recover, they must "drop the rock." After shoveling for hours in the hot sun, sweating, heaving, crying, yelling at anyone who tried to approach, I finally felt a massive cinch in my back, forcing me to rest. I sat there with that shovel, bent over in pain, and when I looked up I saw what I was failing to feel: serenity. It was a warm afternoon, and I could see the sun getting ready to set as a light breeze swept through the great oaks and settled quietly around me. Observing where the staff and clients were going about their business, I beheld our property. The buildings were painted a soft yellow, enclosed by white picket fences; our quaintly painted trash cans depicted landscapes and pictures of animals; and the beauty of our work overcame me. Though people should do what they say they are going to do, I didn't have to make it personal. I didn't need to embarrass John or myself in order to get the emotion across. Like many things in my life, it wasn't about the feeling itself; it was about how I chose to go through it. I became aware of how that anger felt, and in recognizing it, and honoring it, I knew it was time to drop the rock.

Since then, I have learned what anger can do for me, channeling that passion into my work, into educating people about eating disorders, into learning how to manage and work with people better. I have realized that when I am feeling angry about something or someone, I need to pause and check where that anger is coming from. Does it have anything to do with the thing or person in question? Or does it have to do with me? Often what I am angry about or trying to change in someone else's life is none of my business. I have to take that energy and focus it on myself, seeing where I can reach out to others for help, or how I might access resources like training or retreats in order to work through whatever issue I am confronting. And sometimes it's just a matter of my dropping that rock and letting go of the results. I have found that I am a much stronger person when I am not spending energy trying to run other people's lives and am instead able to use that energy to help people when they need and want my help.

As you look at that new self-concept, see where you can do the same. What in your life are you holding on to? What shovel do you need to put down? How can you begin to mind your own business when a situation does not involve you? And, at the same time, where in your life can you affect real and productive change?

The secret to all of this is simple: It starts with you. It is not about changing the world, your family, or your spouse. It's about finding where change needs to take place within you. Looking over your new self-concept, recognize where you can take action today. How can you reach out to another person for help? And what changes need to be made in your behavior and belief systems so that you are able to declare in a safe and respectful way when you have been angered by something? How can you find a solution for that anger, rather than being an accomplice to its rage? See where that energy can propel you into recovery, into exercise, into healthy eating habits, and into the changes that need to take place for an honest and well-lived life.

PROTECTION

The night before Margaret was to leave, she sneaked out of the residential house and decided to go for a walk. Many evenings when I come home from an off-site meeting or errand, I will drive around our neighborhood, looking at how our small community continues to grow: the new shops, my friend's bougainvillea. Sometimes I just drive lost in thought, taking that time in the car as a moment to reflect, and at that moment I was reflecting on Margaret. Her story was so much like my own—an alcoholic mother, an abusive father, and a husband she had managed to love through his alcoholism and recovery. And just as I had, she stood on the precipice of healing, seeing in it a glimmer of hope, but at the same time she was pulled back by her own fear. I turned the corner to head home, my headlights blinding a lone woman walking down the road: Margaret.

I pulled up to her and rolled down my window. "Out for a walk?"

Margaret nodded, knowing that she was supposed to be at the house with the other clients, working on their final journal exercises. I left the car running, the headlights on, and got out, breathing in the cool night air.

"Margaret, you don't need to be afraid of me, of you, or your future."

"I'm sorry, Tennie. But I can't help it. I've been afraid my whole life."

Growing up in similar violence, Margaret spoke my old language of fear. "Come here." I took her hand and led her in front of my car.

"Where are we going?" she asked, already nervous.

"Nowhere—we're staying right here. I want you to stand in front of this car. As you can see, it's running; in fact, it has the power to kill you, right?"

"Yes, so why are we standing in front of it?"

"Because we can. We have faith that it's in park, that it's not going anywhere. It is there to help us, to drive us where we need to go when we ask it to, and we are cautious with it so that we don't get hurt. We have faith that we can be in it every day, and though there might be the occasional accident, the threat of something much worse, we do it, don't we?"

Margaret began to chuckle. "I practically live in mine."

"Right, so do I. Now look behind you." Margaret turned to where her shadow spread out across the pavement, the headlights casting an eerie figure.

"That's what you live in fear of, Margaret. Not the real threat, not the scary five-thousand-pound monster made of metal. You fear the shadow of your past, of your old ideas, of this belief that you're hopeless, and that any change you try to make will fail."

Margaret nodded, tears coming to her eyes. I took her hand. "I understand. I spent my whole life running from that shadow, and it is terrifying. We can't touch it, we can't catch it, and we think that's what makes it so powerful. But the truth is, that's just the evidence that it's not real. It doesn't exist anymore. The past is gone, and that doesn't mean we ignore it, but we stop treating it like a real threat. Because how can we avoid the oncoming cars if we're too busy looking behind us at our shadows?"

"Tennie," Margaret asked, "how did you find me?"

I smiled. "Find you? Heck, I wasn't even looking. I was just out for a drive. Now come on; let me get you back."

There are no coincidences, no mistakes. The spirit of the universe creates miracles for all of us if we are willing to see them, if we can finally stop obsessing about that shadow. We engage in tasks every day that could kill us in an instant, yet we believe that by making the right choices, following a certain set of guidelines, we will be protected. There is no difference between the road to the grocery store and the road to recovery. Though there will always be obstacles—birthday parties, holiday dinners, bad days—we can get wherever we need to go by having faith that God will guide us there. Just as God guided me that night to Margaret. She was so lost in doubt, she couldn't see that faith was just on the other side, begging for her to walk through that shadowy valley of "can't do it" and into the safe and loving arms of the universe.

There is no feeling more powerful than embracing fear. We step into that shadow, and we find that we can hold it with love and faith in God's protection. As you build that new self-concept, see where you can be better guided by faith, opening yourself up to the wisdom it offers. Where do you have fear in your life now? What does that shadow look like, and how can you turn it over to your higher power? How would you like to practice faith in your new self-concept, and where does God fit in? In taking the time to feel our fears, playing out the tape of their possibility and likelihood, we can recognize where God's protection is available to us. What fears are real, and how can you respond to them? Which are false, and what steps can you take on a daily basis in order to let them go? What lessons can be gained from fear, and how can they be applied to your life in this moment?

GROWTH

As Khalil Gibran wrote, "Much of your pain is . . . the bitter potion by which the physician within you heals your sick self." As hard it is to accept, pain is the prescription for healing, demanding that we endure its nauseating side effects in order to be relieved of our symptoms. We can stay in the behaviors, but pain, when great enough, will finally force us out, pushing us to grow.

Stephanie stood in front of the other clients and families who were gathered at Shades for Family Week. She is a tall brunette whose height and weight (three hundred pounds at five-eleven) make for a striking combination, but despite her smoothed-back hair and heavy application of makeup, her weariness was plain. Her father and husband were there, watching as she looked down at one of the other clients, Jane, who was participating in her family sculpt. Jane portrayed Stephanie's mother, who passed away nearly fifteen years before, just as Stephanie was beginning her foray into alcoholism. By the time her mother died, Stephanie was a full-blown alcoholic. Having already been an overeater since childhood, for years she drank and ate, trying not to feel her loss, or the guilt of her inability to show up for her mother or father in their time of need.

Stephanie knelt down by Jane, who lay there, covered by a sheet, representing her mother's death. Stephanie spoke, quietly weeping. "I remember right before you died, you opened your arms really wide and said, 'Enjoy, enjoy, enjoy.' Mother, I'm so sorry. I'm sorry I didn't listen to you. I didn't think I had a right to enjoy; instead I hid from everything. I couldn't grieve, so I stopped feeling altogether. I just want to feel again."

Her father wept from the sidelines as Stephanie laid her head down on Jane's chest, crying out all those years of grief, which had driven her deeper into addiction. Finally Jane put her arms around Stephanie, reacting as though she were her mother, whispering, "Darling, it's time to move on. It's time for you to finally be happy."

Stephanie later told her father that she wanted to enjoy, enjoy, enjoy, but she knew that she could not get there until she was first willing to swallow the bitter pill of pain, allowing herself the tears and grief that the alcohol and food had made inaccessible, even when she finally wanted to feel.

Many food addicts do not allow themselves to feel pain, instead eating it away, pretending it's not there, but it is. It is always there, and we cannot heal without it. We are forever stalled, like Stephanie's grief, unable to process any emotion because we fear going through the pain that life demands, creating one of the biggest obstacles to growth. But as Deirdre, our client who came in drinking a bottle of castor oil every day, once said, "When we allow the pain to pass, we grow spiritually."

So much of this work should take place within a support group or in therapy, but take this time to see where you are ready to grow today. What events or experiences do you want to finally heal from? What pains still linger? How are they disguised by your addictions, unresolved because you haven't wanted to face them? How can your new self-concept begin to process this pain? What do you need in order to finally grieve, recognizing the pain when it comes up and giving yourself the space and time to move through it? How can you find a way to grow from it; what lessons does it offer? How can you handle pain in the future, creating safe boundaries to process the hurt while being open to its message?

Invite your God into this work. Ask Him or Her or It to help you carry that pain. Be still and know that you can embrace it, receiving the gift of growth from its results.

REACHING OUT

The first day Cat arrived, she settled in like a member of the family, comfortable with the other clients, chatting merrily, as though she had always been there. She greeted me with a warm hug, and was open and engaged with all the staff. Cat was in her early thirties at the time, a beautiful and successful writer. But as we continued deeper into her work, we realized that this woman, who acted like a social butterfly among the group, was actually desperately, desperately alone.

Though she was part of a cosmopolitan arts scene in San Francisco, attending all the right cocktail parties and eating at high-end restaurants, navigating professional and social environments with ease and grace, she didn't know how to truly open up to people. Unable to relax that well-developed facade, she couldn't allow herself to be vulnerable. Cat had always "taken care of herself" and, admittedly, didn't know how to reach out to other people, believing that as long as she smiled and laughed, playing the part, they would never know the real Cat: a lonely bulimic who spent her nights and weekends at home bingeing and purging, locked in a hell of her own making.

Her "friends" didn't know, and over the years she had distanced herself from her family as well. Though she had been seeing a therapist for years, she didn't mention it to him either until she started throwing up blood, prompting him to refer her to our six-week residential program at Shades. She listened, arriving less than a week later.

It was on her third week that Cat's facade finally cracked. She had made plenty of friends, including the staff, who adored her, charmed by her easygoing attitude and her sense of humor. One morning at our staff meeting, her primary counselor told us that for as many friends as she was making, as comfortable and happy as she seemed, she had not been doing any of her work, refusing to do the exercises, including her life history.

Around that time, Cat's roommates had requested to see the latest hit movie, which had just come out on DVD. All clients must put in a request for such a privilege, and the whole group had gotten together, including Cat, and had written us a rather creative bid. The outside world feels like a special, almost exotic place when you are living in treatment, devoid of transportation, looking at the same rooms, same road, and same people every day. A movie takes you away for a bit, reminding you of the world in which you live and the one you will soon be returning to. We knew the request meant a lot to the group, and we knew they would be disappointed if we didn't say yes, so we acquiesced under one condition: Cat had to write her life history.

I called Cat into my office to explain the scenario, and I watched that friendly, charming woman just fold up into herself.

"I'm doing the work," she replied. "I go to all the meetings and group sessions and—"

I interrupted. "Look, Cat, I am not here to waste your time, and I doubt you want to waste mine, but if you think we're running a sorority, a six-week stay at Camp Shades, you've come to the wrong place. We're here to save your life, but not if you won't help us. Now, you can play your extrovert role, hiding that shy little girl inside by trying to overcompensate, befriending everyone in Texas, or you can start letting people in."

Peer pressure can be a magical thing when used positively. When the group saw that Cat needed help, they began walking her through it. Showing her their own life histories, they shared how they got through remembering all those terrible tragedies of their pasts. And then Cat began to share her own history—how she was always talked down to as a child, criticized for her weight, her looks, how she dressed. She believed that if only she were thinner, prettier, more outgoing, she might feel better. Finally, it came her turn to share her life story at Family Week in front of her mother and grandmother, who passed along that message that somehow she would never measure up. She shared in front of everyone, "Looking back, I don't remember a time when I wasn't sad. I always felt that sense of loneliness, preferring to play in safe, small, enclosed rooms and little spaces. With the food, either by bingeing or purging, I felt like I was in that safe place, because mentally I would just leave when I was bingeing, and especially when I was purging. Either I was talking to everyone or I was hiding from them, not knowing how to be me. There was never balance, just that sense of desperation."

There is no better way to embrace loneliness than to find a group of people who understand what it means to be lonely. Ultimately, Cat found a program of recovery in which she discovered the honest love and laughter she was only imitating elsewhere in her life. She told me later that she is always mindful of how easily she can still isolate, working one day at a time on staving off loneliness, and learning to find comfort in herself through reaching out to others.

As you reflect on your self-concept, see where you are lonely in your life today. Where and how do you isolate, and how can you begin to change that? There are twelve-step programs for food addicts of all types—overeaters, anorexics, and bulimics—in nearly every city. In those programs you will find a fellowship that can understand and uplift you. Would you like to reach out to one today? Is there another group that you can participate in—one that speaks to your needs and concerns—and are you ready to take that first step, make that phone call? Though at first the phone might feel like it weighs four hundred pounds, the more you get used to reaching out, the more natural it will become. Are you willing to let go of the isolation and helplessness that have kept you in your kitchen, your bathroom, your head stuck in the refrigerator, looking for something you cannot find?

HUMANITY

By the first grade, I had developed a speech impediment that would haunt me throughout childhood. Unable to say my Rs, I was teased mercilessly by my sister, classmates, even my father, who used to force me to ask his friends whether they wanted a glass of water. Tongue-tied, yet still obedient, I would stand in front of the guest and, after much stammering, manage to get out, "Would you like a glass of wataaaa?" Daddy and his friends would laugh until they cried. Eventually my impediment got so bad I was put in a special-education class, which in those days lumped the special-needs children all together. One student in my class was confined to a wheelchair, afflicted with hydrocephalus, a buildup of fluid inside the skull, which leads the brain to swell (then we just called it "water on the brain"). When my sister found out about the handicapped child she began tormenting me in earnest. "Your head is too big for your body," she told me gleefully, adding, "I'll bet you've got water in there, too."

Shame followed me wherever I went: I faced it on the playground, in my living room, and most especially when I looked in the mirror and saw that heavy child with a terrible stutter staring back at me. For years, long after the stutter had left and my sister forgot the boy with the wet brain, I would still look in the mirror and feel the same worthlessness that I did in first grade. It didn't matter what happened in my life, even how much I weighed; I had become frozen in my body. I was fixed in what I thought I could and could not do, always underestimating my abilities.

When I got to treatment, my shame was visceral. Since I was finally being asked to be myself, to be vulnerable and raw in front of complete strangers (though there were only two other clients in my program at the beginning), I just shut down, sinking deeper into that self-hatred, refusing to participate in anything where I had to move my body. So they made me play Ping-Pong, deciding that part of my treatment would be to ask someone every day to play table tennis with me—clients, counselors, even the kitchen staff. At first it was terrifying—having to move around, chasing the ball, watching it roll out of arm's length and having to stretch and move my body in front of someone else to get it. I was embarrassed every time I missed the volley or failed to get it over the net, but then I saw that the other person was having just as many difficulties. After the first week, I started to win a few, gaining confidence and seeing that, like anything in life, the more I did it, the better I got.

Just as it became easier for me to ask someone to join me in the game, so it became easier for me when I had a terrible shot, watching the ball bounce into a far corner, forcing me to run in order to retrieve it. Likewise, it became easier for me to win, to acknowledge my success. I began to see where I did have value, how I could take control of a game, make the winning shot, and still be gracious to the loser. I began to make friends over that silly game of Ping-Pong, which in the end was one of my first lessons in being human. God had not made me so special or unique that I couldn't participate in life. I was just as blessed and able as anyone else. I was not only capable of winning in Ping-Pong, but I could also commit to a meal plan that worked. I could give up years of bingeing and purging for healthy eating, and start entering all of my relationships with humility and humanity.

As you develop your new self-concept, see where you can begin embracing shame, replacing that sense of worthlessness with a deep and powerful humanity. What can you do to begin exercising that humanity? Is there a new way in which you can engage others? Are there boundaries you need to create in order to protect yourself while still allowing others in? How can you invite folks into your life, either through work or play? Can you start creating friendships around your hobbies, asking your family to join you in something you love to do, or joining them in their passions? How can you begin to respect your body through motion, dance, and play, letting go of what you can and cannot do? What can you do today to set yourself free? Is there somewhere in your life where you need to exhibit more humility, watching for the areas in which we overcompensate for our insecurities? Are there certain behaviors that need to be changed or transformed to create more harmony or balance? Shame is the idea that we are everything or nothing, the hero or a zero. But in seeing our humanity, we can appreciate our talents and our flaws. Balance is there for all of us, even if it might look like that Ping-Pong ball, bouncing out of reach.

AMENDS

When Jenny came into Shades, she was raising twins in a wealthy suburb of Atlanta, had been recently divorced from her husband of ten years, and weighed less than ninety pounds. She was so frail, it was hard to imagine her taking care of herself, let alone two third graders, but Jenny had a will that could knock down buildings. She was determined that as long as she kept moving, she would be able to maintain her responsibilities and lifestyle.

On Jenny's fourth day, as she began filling out all the things she was powerless over, and how her eating disorders had made her life unmanageable, she got up from her group session and went to her room. Less than fifteen minutes later, she emerged with her rolling suitcase traveling behind her. I was at home when I received the call that Jenny had left the facility. She stopped by the administrative office and told Cam she was leaving and that any forms or bills could be sent to her later. Knowing there weren't many places for her to go, our staff watched as she walked out the front door, wheeling her way down the lone road out of Shades. Unfortunately for Jenny, she had to roll past my house before she got very far. I had already received the call that she was coming, so I walked outside, prepared to greet her.

She saw me and immediately wagged her finger. "I'm leaving, Mrs. McCarty; you people can't stop me."

"I know that, although there aren't many taxis around here. Where are you planning to walk to?"

"I'll figure it out."

"You always do, don't you?"

She glared at me. "I'm not sick; I don't have a disease."

"Really, well, what's wrong with you, then? Because what I see is a woman who looks like a little girl just lost in her body. And you might be a wonderful mother; I have no doubt you love your children—so much that I am sure you wouldn't have considered leaving them to come here unless you really had to."

Jenny had been suffering from bulimia and anorexia for years, including the time she was pregnant. She had written as much on the client questionnaire that everyone fills out before coming to Shades, and I could see that guilt just washing over her, making her feel that there was no way out, utterly immobilized by her behaviors.

"If you want to make it right by those babies, you shouldn't be going home right now."

Jenny looked at me, stoic despite the pain I could see in her eyes. "I hurt them, you know. I was so sick during the pregnancies that they ended up being born underweight. They both still suffer from breathing issues, and when I told the doctor what had happened, he said it was my fault, that I had caused their complications."

"I know, baby. I know you walk around with that every day, dragging it like that suitcase there, but turning your back on this program, on this chance to do things differently, is just going to make it more likely that you will repeat the things you've already done. We cannot change the past, but we can mend it."

There was no doubt that the choices she had made were terrible and their consequences heartbreaking, but the guilt was far worse. The negative case she had made against herself was so powerfully amplified that she thought she would die from it, and she almost did.

That day Jenny rolled her way back to Shades, and back to the work that ultimately set her free, relieving her of the burden she had carried for so long. She began to have hope, seeing where she could have a new chance at life and at motherhood. Though she was anxious to heal the relationship with her family, she later told me, "I learned that it wasn't about my being crazy or wounded; it was about getting healed so I could transfer that healing to my life and my family."

As you look at your self-concept, see where you need to forgive yourself. Where are you harboring guilt in your life today, immobilized by its presence? What first steps can you do to break out of it, working toward self-forgiveness before you ask others to forgive? As you assess your value system, what changes need to be made to reflect who you are today? And do you need to make changes to your boundaries to stay in line with those values? Where are you carrying guilt that isn't yours or is exaggerated past the point of its reality? Whom have you injured, or where do things need to be set right? There are few harms in this world that cannot be undone. For the most part, we can always mend what is broken. We can stop beating ourselves up and finally get off our own backs. As we begin to share this guilt with others, we will find that we are not such bad human beings after all; we are simply human. We make mistakes, we right those mistakes, and, in redeveloping our value system, we create new behaviors.

Hope

I remember years ago, when my Al-Anon mentor Anne started teaching me how to have fun, she was instructing me in something I had never done. This was years before I went into treatment for my own disorders. At the time, I had joined Al-Anon to "fix" RL's alcoholism, thinking that if I entered a program of recovery, so might he. Unfortunately, Anne wasn't interested in getting RL healthy; she was more interested in my mental state.

"I want you to follow this schedule," Anne told me. "It's simple: eight hours of work, eight hours of play, and eight hours of rest."

Though I thought she was half loony, I decided to follow her advice. I started taking the early afternoons for myself, trying to do something other than clean the house or eat from the kitchen. One day, not long into my experiment, RL came home to find me sitting in a lounge chair at the side of our pool, getting a tan.

"How was your day?" I asked as he approached me, sensing his frustration from a distance.

"What in the hell are you doing?"

"I'm getting some sun," I replied.

"Ever since you started going to those damn Al-Anon meetings you've become indifferent," he complained. "You no longer wash my pickup, and you don't even wash your own car. You don't mow the grass or do the yard. Instead you've hired other people to do your work."

Though I tease him about it today, he really said that. My husband and children were so used to my being their secretary, housekeeper, and servant that they didn't know what do with the new me. They were accustomed to a mother who was like a whirling dervish, rushing from one chore to the next. But in teaching my then teenaged children to do their own darn laundry, I began to taste what joy could feel like. I soaked in the sun and, reveling in the spirit of God, I received hope that one day I might heal. And I began to let go of the idea that RL had to.

I ask that you begin to make the same schedule for yourself. Create days where you give yourself eight hours of work, eight hours of play, and eight hours of rest. In your new self-concept, what would that play look like? How would you spend your time if you could? Don't just turn on the TV and call that "play." Play is getting out and going for a walk, doing your nails, playing basketball, going to the gym—moving and treating yourself with love and respect. How can you have fun today? As you finish up that self-concept, list the hobbies you have always wished to begin, the promises and resolutions of a more active life that you know would bring you joy if you could only do them, and stopped dreaming about them. Describe yourself with all of these elements of play present in your life—what will you be like, and how will you grow?

It was through Snoopy that I found my concept of God, and I have seen similar rediscoveries of God happen for so many others. Once we allow that inner child to come out, that little girl or boy begins to do some of the directing, and we begin to find out who we really are. Our divine self, the part of us that is most connected to the will of the universe, is now the one in charge. We find the one thing we love outside of our addiction, and our mission becomes apparent. This mission doesn't always have to be our profession; however, if you want to go out and make your passion your career, by all means do it—that's what I did. But we can also realize that mission through our hobbies, through volunteer work, and through our relationships.

The Power of Affirmations

I remember back in the 1990s when *Saturday Night Live* had that wonderful Stuart Smalley skit of affirmations: "I'm good enough, I'm smart enough, and, doggone it, people like me." I was in the middle of the recovery movement at that time, and though most of us had a sense of humor about it, we had also seen how transformational those affirmations could be.

The brain is the most magnificent computer ever made, capable of being rewired and reprogrammed just like any PC or Mac on the market. Affirmations are the programmer, reinforcing a chemical pathway in the brain wherein the connection between two neurons is made stronger and more likely to reproduce that message we have just offered ourselves. Neurologists like to say that "neurons that fire together wire together." These neurons form a pattern that is strengthened by repetition. If we hear repeated negative messages, it is those messages that will determine the pattern; if we hear positive ones, they will alternatively become embedded in our psyche, forming a new basis for our belief system.

We literally create a new tape, a new system of messaging in our neural passageways, which is founded on positive reinforcement—about how we are beautiful, how we are loved, and how we are deserving of change. Every day at Shades, staff and clients stand up after every meal, offering five affirmations about their body and life, rewiring their thinking to establish that new self-concept. No one immediately believes the words they are saying (we are trying to overturn decades of bad messaging here), but the more they speak these positive affirmations, the more they begin to believe in their power to change. The affirmations must be positive, they must be in the present, and they must be precise—short enough to state in one brief sentence. Folks will say things like:

- I love my stomach.
- My thighs are beautiful.
- I am a good mother.
- I appreciate my family.
- I am grateful for my eyes.

Review your self-concept, which should now be complete, identifying fifty affirmations from your description. Take those goals, those promises to yourself, and turn them into positive, present, and precise statements that you can use to affirm this new tape, revising those messages you took in so long ago. I have been doing it for decades, standing in front of the mirror and offering myself varying resolutions of self-love, faith, and inspiration. I know it can be embarrassing, but I also know it can change your life. Write them on Post-its, and attach them to your bathroom mirror, your computer, your closet, or even in your car. I removed one of the mirrors from a double compact, slipping in a short list of affirmations so that I could repeat them at any time and anywhere. Find the easiest and most convenient way to make them a part of your life, and you will see what science has proved: that you can alter how you perceive yourself, taking that new self-concept and making it real.

After you have written your list, double-check to make sure it is positive. The affirmations should never be insulting or negative. There are no *no*s in affirming. They should only complement you and your progress. Once you have them ready, go to a mirror, look at yourself in the pupils, and repeat them one at a time. Start today and give yourself two weeks, journaling your changes so that you can be watchful of and present for your growth.

TWELVE

Meal Plan

*P*aula stood up at the dining room table, ready to repeat her affirmations, beginning with the one that is repeated at Shades more than any other: "Just for today, I am going to do what is good, right, and honest for my body and in my life."

As she said "my body," she began to cry, sitting back down, unable to continue.

No one said anything; they were, at that point, accustomed to letting folks go through their emotions. We don't try to console, or interrupt their course. In fact, to the outside world, we might even look a little rude, refraining from handing the person a tissue or rubbing his or her back. But our society is structured around this idea that comfort should quell pain. And it does. It absolutely disrupts the pain process, pulling people out of the emotion before they can successfully complete it. It's like that movie *The Matrix*, where the characters would be in their other world, intent on completing a mission, but at any moment the folks back on the mother ship could cut the cord to that reality, returning them to the present. And we do need to come back to the present. Our whole goal is to live in that present, but we can't very well do that if our mission has been cut short, leaving us neither here nor there.

Finally I asked Paula, "Where are the tears coming from?"

"I just can't believe I'm here again."

This wasn't Paula's first round at Shades of Hope. Ten years prior, she came in forty pounds underweight, a chronic anorexic who knew only how to starve. But then Paula healed; she gained back the weight, returning home to a recovery program and a conscious and consistent meal plan. She went on to graduate college, found a career, and not long afterward she got married and had a family. After the birth of her first son, she started to go off her meal plan and cut back on her meetings, and over time she found herself on the other side of the scale: sixty pounds overweight.

Paula sat there in baby blue sweats that had grown too tight, her black hair pulled back in a bun, and her otherwise delicate features swollen from the food and the tears. She confessed, "I never thought that this is what I would look like. I don't ever want to go back to being that stick person, but this is just as bad. Why do I have such problems with food?"

Why do I have such problems with food? Research is beginning to prove what many eating-disorder professionals have been saying all along: Food addiction is a disease and should be treated like a disease. In 1994 UCLA conducted a study discovering that some obese adults had the same D2 dopamine gene marker that distinguished alcoholism and drug addiction, even if the adult in question was not addicted to either chemical substance. Furthering that theory, a recent research program in France showed that "intense sweetness"—not just refined sugar, but also artificial sweeteners—surpasses cocaine as a reward in laboratory animals.

For many folks with eating disorders, this "problem with food" has little or nothing to do with willpower, and everything to do with chemical dependency. Some of us are emotional eaters, relying on food for that comfort that can so easily remove us from our feelings. Others are addicted to the physical components of sugar, white flour, or even wheat. But often the food addict struggles with both, confounded by the two-fold illness of addiction. Thus far, we have seen how we can respond with a spiritual and emotional solution: finding a God of our understanding and finally allowing ourselves the emotional processing we have made a habit of interrupting. But the crucial piece in all of this is how we respond to the physical cravings. How do we train that tiger so that we may bring him out of his cage and take him on his walk without finding ourselves back at the dinner table, sixty pounds overweight, wondering why we have such problems with food?

Taking the Feelings Out of Food

As Paula sat there, staring down at the tablecloth, I could see in her the defeat I have seen in so many others addicted to their plates, and involuntarily going back for more. They want what they want when they want it—even when they don't want it anymore.

"Paula, when was the last time you followed your meal plan?"

She sniffed back the tears. "It's not that."

"Oh, it's not? What is it, then?"

"I don't know—I went to the doctor, thinking maybe it was a thyroid problem. I even started going to a nutritionist."

"Well, that's all good stuff, but you didn't answer the question. When was the last time you followed your meal plan?"

She glared at me. "I have children, a husband, and they want certain foods that aren't on the plan. I should be able to participate in meals with my family. I should be able to control what I eat without a stupid plan."

When I came home from treatment, I had no idea how I was going to make my whole family eat what I ate. I was convinced that we would never have Thanksgiving again, and I would be consigned to a lifetime of eating by myself at the corner table. But I discovered how far from the truth that was; healthy eating is for everyone, and often our families need it just as much as we do.

"That is bull, Paula. That is bull and you know it. It is the disease offering you that excuse." I looked around the table at all the other clients as I continued. "We need that meal plan like a diabetic needs his or her insulin. It teaches us how to eat safely, and there is nothing about it that excludes our family. I can make meals for everyone in my household, hosting the holidays while still keeping to my plan, but what I can't do is eat healthy without it. In setting my physical boundaries around food, I can hopefully be an example to others."

In order for us to take the feelings out of our food, to keep our plate entirely objective so that it doesn't reflect anything back to us other than the meal upon it, we must be on a food plan. We must be conscious in every choice, in every measurement, watching what we buy, what we cook, what we eat, and how often those meals take place. To think that there is any other way is to be conned by the disease.

Paula tried to avoid my attention, fiddling with her fork.

"Paula, stop playing with the fork; don't you think you've done that enough? You almost died because of this disease. You thought that you had to maintain control, while you had nothing even close to it. And you're doing the same thing again, thinking you should be able to control your eating. The meal plan removes us from that whole process, takes us out of the equation of control, but I'm wondering: Are you ready to surrender?"

The question is the same for you. Are you ready to surrender? Are you absolutely exhausted by the endless diets and disappointment, by the overextension that controlling your life demands, by being addicted to what is on your plate?

THE END OF THE EXCUSE

For years, we have lived in all the reasons a healthy meal plan will not work. We tell ourselves we don't have time. We explain that it's too difficult when we have a full-time job or we're feeding a family. We fall back on our childhoods or the people we like to blame for the misery we are now creating. But underneath all these excuses is nothing but plain old fear. Once you get rid of the reasons why not, you need to explore how to.

As you look at this work, what is your recovery going to look like? Do you plan to join a twelve-step group? Do you intend to work the meal plan? Have you completed the exercises in this book? Have you begun to think that treatment might be the solution? What do you want your abstinence to look like, and how do you plan on achieving it? Go ahead and write a page about what you want to commit to in order to be free of your addiction to food.

Then look over that plan and see what excuses stand between you and its realization. Write each excuse down on its own piece of paper. At Shades, we burn those sheets, eliminating them from our realities. But tearing them up and throwing them in the trash will do just as well. Read each one aloud, and hear how ridiculous it sounds. Decide whether those excuses are worth more than your life. And then tear them into pieces and make the commitment to your abstinence, removing all the obstacles from its attainment.

Abstinent Eating

Food addiction is just like any other addiction, producing cravings we cannot control, driving us to eat. The Food Addiction Institute, an educational organization dedicated to the research and wider understanding of this epidemic, offers, "Fifteen years ago there were less than a dozen articles on food addiction. . . . Today there are 2,748 peer-reviewed journal articles and books related to food as a chemical dependency." This dependency is best characterized as a cluster of physical reactions. The institute continues, "Just like there are several different drugs that can be addictive, there are several different foods—and sometimes food in general—that can be addictive."

By identifying the chemicals upon which you are dependent (sugar, flour, excessive fats, wheat, or caffeine), you are able to define your abstinence. The best test for this is to try to abstain from each for one week, watching how your body responds, and seeing whether withdrawals occur. If you experience withdrawals from a specific chemical, you can be sure you are addicted.

If you are addicted to one of the above, it is strongly suggested you remove it from your meal plan, abstaining from it for a full year as you build and develop your sound and sober eating practices. If after that time, you want to see whether you can eat it in balance, then you can give it a try. Some people can add sugar, caffeine, limited fats, and flour back into their diets in moderation, and some cannot. The key to abstinent eating is that we don't do it alone. You need to hire a nutritionist or enter a program of recovery wherein you can find a food sponsor to help you design your food plan and stay within its boundaries.

That's not to say you won't make mistakes. Falling off the plan is not a sin. It has no bearing on your value or your ability to ultimately maintain the plan. Most addicts like to think, *I'm a good girl (or a good boy), and I have to do it perfectly. If I make one mistake, I've blown it, and I might as well go back to eating as I like.* This is where the addict needs to change, learning to live in the gray zone of healthy eating, being conscious of her decisions, and gentle with herself.

The meal plan is our course and we set out on it, but if we stray, we return to the path without beating ourselves up. We get off our own backs, forgiving our mistakes and recommitting to our recovery. That doesn't mean it will be easy. As Paula saw, once she got off the meal plan, she created an opening for her old thinking to return, convincing her that she didn't need it, that the solution lay elsewhere.

The four secrets to eating sober are simple:

1. Moderation—Portion control is the guiding factor of any healthy meal plan. What we eat is important, but how much we eat is what determines addictive versus nonaddictive behavior. We must uphold moderation in our food, eating for nutritional value, and no longer for emotional comfort.

2. Variety—So many diets fail in one area: They have no variety. We cannot be expected to eat the same things over and over and enjoy the results. We need to keep variety in our meal plan, never allowing for the same meal or food item more than three times a week. Likewise, we also limit how often we go out to eat. There are plenty of safe foods at almost any restaurant in the country, but we do not need to go out to eat more than three times a week. We need to create a meal plan that engages us, that includes many foods we like and love, and that offers us the variety we need in order to maintain it.

3. Balance—This goes back to that good girl/bad boy concept. We aim to stay committed to our meal plan for a full year, but we do not throw it all away because of one slip, but rather recommit to our plan if we do fall off. By seeking balance in our diet, living in the gray area that abstinence demands, we will be able to bring balance to the rest of our lives. It is not about perfection; it is about progress.

4. Hydration—Seventy-five percent of Americans are chronically dehydrated, and in 37 percent of Americans the thirst mechanism is so weak that being thirsty is often mistaken for hunger.

Water is one of the most important sources of life on our planet, critical to our chemistry, our environment, and our health. In order to eat healthy, you must drink healthy—consuming at least sixty-four ounces of water each day. Though we may add two nonwater beverages a day, they in no way replace the nutritional value of water. Diet Coke is not H_2O. I know I am not the first to offer this suggestion, but by staying hydrated you will no longer confuse thirst for hunger.

Nutrition is available to all of us. We don't need to cut everything from our diet; nor do we need to play tricky games to eat right. It is not about dieting; it is about eating abstinent, healthy meals that provide us with nutrients to move through our day. They are meals that can be made and served to the whole family, creating healthy eating habits for everyone in our life.

We cannot manipulate a meal plan. It won't listen to our excuses or rationalizations. It is immune to the tricks our addictive minds like to play. By sticking to the plan, we are able to do what is good, right, and honest for our bodies and in our lives. There is no guessing game to healthy eating, only guidelines that, if followed, will lead you to abstinence.

The Plan

The Shades of Hope food plan has been developed to specifically meet the nutritional needs of the recovering food addict. It is based on the U.S. Dietary Guidelines for healthy eating, and incorporates the latest findings concerning abstinence and food addiction, providing for abstinent living, gradual weight loss—or gain, for those under their healthy weight—and well-balanced nutrition.

When folks come into Shades, they meet with a nutritionist, who determines whether there are any additions or subtractions that need to be made to the plan before they start. But with only a few exceptions, almost everyone is on the same plan. That is because this is a plan not based on how much you want to eat, but on what your body needs to be productive and useful throughout the day. At first, everyone feels hungry from it. Most people have been consuming more calories than they would ever need, for years. And when they start eating the amount they actually need, that gap between what was and what is can feel insurmountable. But it's not.

After they get past the first week, most people say the same thing: "I feel amazing." Because our bodies want to be healthy. They don't want to be expending energy trying to burn off calories that aren't necessary. They are efficient machines that prefer to be used efficiently, and once we start eating healthy, the body responds. People feel lighter, happier, experiencing a new sense of freedom just by releasing themselves from the burden of food.

Give yourself a week. Work with friends as you start the process. Go to your journal and write down every night how you are feeling, and you, too, will see the transformation. You will finally experience what it means to feel physically well.

To begin, you should consult a nutritionist or doctor to identify your maintenance weight, based on your height, body type, and nutritional needs. As you approach that weight, you should check back with your physician, dietician, or food sponsor for guidance to adjust your food plan for maintenance. If you are under the care of a physician for any medical problem, you should have your physician review this food plan to make sure that it meets all your dietary needs.

Most food addicts have spent their lives counting calories and memorizing nutritional information, treating it like money in the bank. They'll spend these calories here and save those there, and somehow they will always be guilty of creative accounting. They buy and sell themselves food, thinking they can make up for it later. This food plan is not about counting calories. We remove the barter from eating, and instead view our diet in terms of the right balance of carbohydrates, protein, fats, vitamins, minerals, fiber, and water. Below are some of the items it is suggested you do without.

SUGAR AND CAFFEINE

Sugar and caffeine are nonnutritive, addictive substances that have been found to elicit cravings in food addicts. According to the Food Addiction Institute, "While there is not yet one gene which marks the difference between those who are hypersensitive to sugar and those who are not, there are many studies which show the brains of those who binge on sweets have defects in serotonin brain receptors, rapid spikes in their blood sugar and a hyperinsulin reaction to food." Though not everyone is addicted to sugar, most people who suffer from an unhealthy relationship to food are also not able to healthily eat and process sugars. *This is why we suggest abstaining from sugar for your first year, and then deciding later whether it is safe for you to return to it in small amounts, under the guidance of a nutritionist or food sponsor.*

As for caffeine, two cups of coffee will cause your body to secrete 80 percent more adrenaline than normal, which in turn lowers blood sugar levels and triggers feelings of hunger and cravings. Some food addicts can drink coffee safely; I know my daughters are certainly able to. But I had such a long and brutal history with caffeine addiction, believing it would suppress my appetite when it only did the opposite, that to this day I still do not drink caffeinated beverages. Again, stop caffeine for a week, and you will quickly see whether you share such a dependency.

ALCOHOL

Alcohol is the sugar by-product of grain fermentation, which is itself a type of sugar and will cause sugar cravings. The Food Addiction Institute reports that "approximately 6–8% of those undergoing bariatric surgery for obesity have a severe drinking problem within a year."

In order to avoid such cross-addiction, substituting one dependency for another, we suggest that alcohol is also abstained from in the first year. For many, they believe that the food addiction is the primary issue, either unaware of or in denial over how much they drink. By removing the alcohol from your diet, you will quickly see whether you have been masking another problem behind the food.

FLOUR AND TRIGGER FOODS

Foods that contain flour have been found to provoke the binge response in food addicts. Though trigger foods vary from individual to individual (some relying more on sugar and sweets, others on heavy carbs such as breads and pasta), they all share the same dangerous quality: triggering a binge by the addict's emotional response to food. Due to the tendency of food made with flour to be eaten in large quantities, and flour's refined nature, it is also eliminated from the food plan.

TEXTURED FOODS

Food addicts typically binge on sweet/smooth or salty/crunchy foods; therefore the consistency of a certain food will trigger the binge response even though the food item is by definition "abstinent." Examples of this are "crunchies"—popcorn, rice cakes, or low-fat chips—or "smoothies"—peanut butter or cream cheese. The goal in recovery is to keep food, whenever possible, in its most whole, unrefined form (i.e., baked potato instead of mashed). This tends to ensure greater satiety and generally higher fiber intake.

FRIED/SALTY FOODS

According to the Food Addiction Institute, "The most recently identified gene marker is H(2), which is related to biological breakdowns of the mechanism for digesting fat. . . . There are whole groups of addicts who have cravings for fat, some of whom—mostly from Mediterranean and African heritages—have little or no problem with sugar." In accordance with the American Heart Association, the meal plan avoids high-fat foods such as bacon, sausage, and fried foods in order to ensure abstinence for the fat addict as well as those struggling with sugar and flour.

Guidelines

When you see your physician, have her review this program, and follow her suggestions concerning any changes or alterations that need to be made based on your health, size, gender, age, and activity level.

This meal plan cannot be done on its own.

If you're like me, you have pretended to be on meal plans and diets enough times in your life, keeping them like a secret so those around you wouldn't know when and whether you failed. In order to properly work a meal plan, you need to find a support group to whom you can be accountable, and who can provide you with the emotional support and collaboration you will need to maintain your abstinence. I know that once I started in a fellowship of people who understood what I had gone through, and met a food sponsor who escorted me along my emotional and spiritual journey, the meal plan was a natural result of the work, and not just another diet created for me to fail at.

Please note that this food plan is higher in fiber, which not only decreases the risk of heart disease and cancer but also stabilizes blood sugar. This has been found to be helpful in the treatment of food addiction, since it encourages fullness, reduces cravings, and produces a natural laxative effect that is helpful in promoting regularity of bowel functions. Though this meal plan includes wheat-based starches, it should be noted that if you have celiac disease, in which your intestines stop working when they are forced to process gluten (most often in the form of wheat, but also corn, barley, and rye), you must exchange all wheat-based starches for a gluten-free option. This will be highlighted in the meal plan, and alternatives are suggested.

Below are some guidelines that, if adhered to, will make the tenets of the meal plan much easier to follow:

- Eat at regular times each day. The maximum time between meals is five hours, except for when sleeping, and the minimum time is four hours (unless you have planned snacks per your nutritionist's suggestion).
- Eat all foods on your meal plan each day, never skipping meals or replacing a food in one category with another. For example, don't swap cottage cheese (a protein) for milk (a dairy).
- Weigh and measure all amounts of specified foods using a diet, digital, or postal scale, measuring cups, or spoons. "Eyeballing" is not accurate.
- Plan ahead by shopping weekly, using a menu as a guide when you make your shopping list. I used to make my menu on Friday, write my list on Saturday, and then shop on Sunday to guarantee that I wasn't shopping from impulse, but rather after thoughtful preparation.
- Include foods in their whole, unrefined form to ensure satiety and adequate fiber, and keep foods simple and separate, with

only occasional use of casseroles, etc. Be creative using herbs and spices, but be sure to avoid too much sodium (salt).

- Fresh and frozen vegetables and fruits are preferable, when possible. Canned vegetables are highest in sodium (and fruits in sugar) and offer the lowest nutritional value.
- Do not use:
  - Sugar—also known as sucrose, corn syrup, corn sweetener, fructose, glucose, maltose, lactose, honey, dextrose, concentrated fruit juices, and molasses syrup. Artificial sweeteners may be used, but no more than three packets per day.
  - Flour, arrowroot or cornstarch, agar, and kudzu
  - Diet candies and puddings
  - Alcohol or condiments containing alcohol (including extracts)
  - Fried foods
  - Specialty cheeses, cream cheeses, or hard cheeses (until you reach your maintenance weight)
- Sit down for meals, remaining seated while you eat gently and slowly. Do not eat meals in front of the TV.
- Do not weigh yourself more than once a month, and if any food becomes a binge or trigger food, leave it out after consulting with a dietician or food sponsor.
- Read all labels. By law, all food must display an ingredient listing even if nutritional information is not available. *When in doubt, leave it out!*
- Remove skin from poultry after cooking; drain fats after browning meats such as beef, and cut off visible fat from all meat. When using vegetarian proteins, you may want to combine them with a meat or cheese, i.e., two ounces of beans per two ounces of shredded cheese or meat.
- Eat only what is on your meal plan, and do not alter the plan without discussing with a dietician or food sponsor.

- Daily meal plans are to be:
  - Planned ahead
  - Written down
  - Called in to a sponsor
  - Eaten in their entirety

Below is the daily food plan for all women. Again, a nutritionist should be advised in case you might need additions to or subtractions from the plan, but it is created to provide the targeted nutritional needs of most women.

Breakfast	Lunch	Dinner	Evening Snack
8 oz. low-fat milk or plain yogurt	½ cup starch	½ cup starch	8 oz. low-fat milk or plain yogurt
	3 oz. protein	3 oz. protein	
1 fruit	1 cup vegetables	1 cup vegetables	1 fruit
1 oz. cereal	1 cup salad	1 cup salad	1 oz. cereal
2 oz. protein	1 fat	1 fat	

For men, the meal plan is as follows:

Breakfast	Lunch	Dinner	Evening Snack
8 oz. low-fat milk or plain yogurt	½ cup starch	1 cup starch	8 oz. low-fat milk or plain yogurt
	4 oz. protein	4 oz. protein	
1 fruit	1 cup vegetables	1 cup vegetables	1 fruit
1 oz. cereal	1 cup salad	1 cup salad	1 oz. cereal
2 oz. protein	1 fat	1 fat	

In addition, both men and women may also consume two eight-ounce servings of a decaf, sugar-free drink each day, and one cup of (sugar-free) clear broth with lunch or dinner.

Going Shopping

Planning is the key to abstinence. It is much easier to eat healthy if you keep to a schedule, always making sure you have your food ready for mealtime. As you prepare your shopping list, identify what some of your favorite foods are, or what foods you might be craving that specific week. For example, if I have a desire for fish and pork, I know that I should create some meals based around those proteins. For fruits I love apples, pomegranates, and oranges, so, likewise, I want to make sure I have plenty of those around. I also think about what my favorite kinds of food are: Chinese, Mexican, and vegetarian. I grew up in west Texas, so there is no separating me from my Mexican food. I just had to learn how to cook it in a healthy way and to stick to the portions allotted.

What does your food list look like?

- Proteins—List your three favorite meats or meat substitutes (chicken, pork, beef, soy meats, tofu).
- Starches—List your three favorite starches (potatoes, bread, yams, etc.).
- Vegetables—List your five favorite vegetables (broccoli, asparagus, cauliflower, etc.).
- Fruit—List your five favorite fruits (cantaloupe, pineapple, pears, etc.).
- Fats—List your three favorite fats (favorite cheeses, oils, nut butters).

- Dairy—List your two favorite types of dairy (what kind of milk/ what kind of yogurt).
- Kinds of food—List your three favorite types of food (Italian, Mexican, etc.).

When food addicts are forced to consider their food, they begin to be mindful about it. They are no longer able to eat with abandon. They create a process around food rather than a compulsion. The beauty of this meal plan is that each individual designs it to his or her liking; it is a design for life. Though everyone around you will not necessarily be on the same meal plan—you might sit down across from your husband or go out to lunch with your coworkers and find them eating a very different meal from you—this isn't about anyone else's food. This is about yours. This isn't about anyone else's body—it's about yours. This isn't about anyone else's life—it is about your life.

Before you begin your meal plan you will need to go out and get yourself a decent food scale and some good measuring utensils in one-cup and half-cup portions. We need to start looking at our food in objective measurements. We are finished eating subjective portions based on our emotional demands; instead we begin weighing our food to meet our nutritional needs.

Food Groups with Selections

Below you will find the exchanges for each food group, with examples of selections from each. Though there are certainly other products on the market that will work just as well, please keep in mind that you must confirm whether they are within the meal plan guidelines, consulting beforehand with a dietician or food sponsor. The best way to do this is to go shopping with that dietician, your sponsor, or even a friend in your support group, identifying what in your marketplace you can and cannot eat in accordance with your diet. Everything in these selections can be found at the most basic of markets, and as you shop, always keep in mind that the healthiest and most unrefined foods are on the perimeter of the store. You want the majority of your shopping to be in a plastic produce bag, not in a cardboard box.

FOOD LIST

The following are the major food groups that are found in the food plan:

Dairy	Cereals	Breakfast Proteins
Fruits	Proteins	Starches
Cooked Vegetables	Salad Greens	Fats
Spices and herbs	Condiments	Beverages

Each of these food groups will be described in detail, with examples of the best foods from each. In working with a nutritionist you might add some items to each food group that are not presented here. If you want something that is not on the list, check with your food sponsor or nutritionist to see whether it can be added. There are always ways to modify your food plan, but they must be done hand in hand with someone else.

Group One—Dairy

For your daily dairy exchanges, you should have:

8 oz. skim or 1 percent milk
8 oz. low-fat, sugar-free yogurt

Group Two—Cereals

For your one ounce of cereal or grain, make sure it is low in sugar by checking on the label that sugar is listed as the fifth ingredient or lower (the ingredients are always listed in decreasing order). Sugar is sugar—when in doubt, leave it out!

HIGH-FIBER CEREALS	GRAINS	OTHERS*
Cornflakes (Grainfield's)	Barley	Puffed corn
Cream of rice	Brown rice	Puffed Kashi
Grape-Nuts	Cream of wheat	Puffed rice
Millet	Kashi	Puffed wheat
Nutri-Grain wheat flakes	Oatmeal	
Oat bran/wheat bran	Rye berries	
Shredded wheat	Wheat berries	
Uncle Sam		
*These cereals are lower in fiber and should not be used as often.		

Group Three—Breakfast Proteins

One large egg is equal to two ounces of protein. No more than four eggs per week are recommended. Although permissible, yogurt is not equivalent to the other proteins on this list and should not be used every day.

Dairy (2 oz.)	Proteins	Others
Feta	Canadian bacon	Egg substitute—2 oz.
Fresh farmer's cheese	Chicken	Eggs—1 large
Low-fat cottage cheese	Fish	Low-fat plain yogurt—2 oz.
Low-fat ricotta cheese	Lean beef	Tempeh—2 oz.
Pot cheese	Turkey	Tofu—2 oz.
Note: Do not use bacon, sausage, cured ham, or any high-fat breakfast meat.		

Group Four—Fruits

Fruit is key to the meal plan and to your satiation. Only extreme sugar addicts need adjust their intake of fruit, and must consult with their food sponsor or dietician to do so. Otherwise, all of the following fruits are recommended for the plan:

1 Cup Fresh Fruit		Fresh Fruit Exception
Apples	Oranges	Apricots—2 small
Blackberries	Peaches	Bananas—1 medium/week
Blueberries	Pears	Grapefruit—½
Cantaloupe	Pineapple	Grapes—½ cup
Cranberries	Raspberries	Kiwi—2 small
Honeydew melon	Strawberries	Nectarines—2 small
Mangoes	Watermelon	Plums—2 small
Mixed fresh fruit		
Note: Do not pack in fruit when measuring—there must be spaces between pieces.		

FROZEN FRUIT—1 CUP		
Blackberries	Cantaloupe	Peaches
Blueberries	Honeydew melon	Raspberries
Boysenberries	Mixed frozen fruit	Strawberries

Frozen fruit must be thawed carefully. To measure accurately, the thawed fruit must be whole, and use frozen fruit that does not have artificial sweeteners, concentrated juices, or added ingredients.

CANNED FRUIT—½ CUP	
Apricots	Peaches
Mandarin oranges	Pears
Mixed canned fruit	Pineapple

Use only canned fruit that is packed in its own juices—no added sweeteners, syrups, or concentrates.

Group Five—Proteins

As listed in the plan, women are to consume three ounces of cooked proteins per identified meal, and four ounces for men. Note the few exceptions under vegetarian proteins.

LEAN PROTEIN	FISH AND SHELLFISH	VEGETARIAN PROTEIN	DAIRY/ CHEESE
Center-cut loin pork chops	Clams	Dried beans: 1 cup protein + 1 cup starch (limit 3 times/week)	Low-fat cottage cheese
Chicken breast	Cod	Tempeh (3 oz. for women; 4 oz. for men)	
Chicken leg	Crab	Tempeh burgers (3 oz. for women; 4 oz. for men)	
Chicken thigh	Lobster	Tofu—cooked weight (6 oz. for women; 8 oz. for men)	
Cubed beef	Mackerel		
Eggs—poached, scrambled or boiled	Mussels		
Fresh ham—not cured	Oysters		
Flank steak	Salmon		
Ground round	Scallops		
Ground sirloin	Shrimp		
Lamb loin chops	Sole		
Roast leg of lamb	Trout		
Round steak	Tuna		
Tenderloin			
Turkey breast			
Whole chicken			
Note: No more than 4 eggs per week. Meats may be baked, broiled, microwaved, or grilled.	*Note: Any fish fillet or steak of your choice.*	*Note: Typically, oil is added to tempeh and tofu when making burgers; therefore, one patty of a tofu or tempeh burger is equivalent to one regular meat burger patty.*	*Note: Do not use hard cheeses until you have reached maintenance weight, and limit to three cheeses per week for protein.*

Group Six—Starches

There is a half-cup allowance of starch for both men and women at lunch, but men are allowed a full cup at dinner. Starch must be measured after cooking, as the raw weight will change in the cooking process. If you have celiac disease and are wheat-intolerant, avoid all wheat grains in order to prevent illness and prevent hunger.

GRAINS	BEANS/PEAS*	OTHERS*
Barley	Black beans	Acorn squash
Brown rice—short or long*	Black-eyed peas	Butternut squash
Buckwheat—grained or instant	Black soybeans	Corn on the cob
Kasha—roasted buckwheat	Chickpeas (also called garbanzo beans)	Cut corn
		Parsnips
Millet	Kidney beans	Potatoes—new, baked or broiled
Oats*	Lentils—red, green, and yellow	*Note: Potatoes should be weighed, not measured—4 oz. for women and 8 oz. for men.*
Rye berries		
Wheat berries	Lima beans	
Note: White rice may be used if brown rice is not available.	Peas—green	
	Split beans—green/yellow/white beans—any kind	

*Gluten-free and celiac-friendly items.
Note: In addition to the meal allowance, when making meat loaf, up to two table-spoons of any grain may be used with one pound of meat.

Group Seven—Cooked Vegetables

Per the meal plan, one cup of cooked vegetables is suggested for both men and women. Vegetables should be mixed, as using a variety of colors will assure a healthy variety of vitamins and minerals. Fresh and frozen vegetables are recommended, but canned may be used. When using raw vegetables in a salad, allow one cup for both men and women. For one meal per day, you may substitute one cup of raw vegetables for one cup of cooked.

VEGETABLES	
Artichokes—1 medium	Chili peppers
Asparagus	Collard greens
Bamboo shoots	Cucumbers
Beans—green, Italian, pole, and wax	Daikon radish
Bell peppers—red, yellow	Dandelion greens*
Beet greens*	Dill pickles
Bok choy	Eggplant
Broccoli*	Kale
Brussels sprouts	Mustard greens*
Cabbage	Okra
Carrot tops	Parsley
Carrots*	Radishes
Cauliflower	Rutabagas
Celery	Sauerkraut
Cherry tomatoes	Scallions

Snow peas (pea pods)	Summer/crookneck squash
Spinach*	Swiss chard—red, green
Sprouts—alfalfa, mung bean	Tomatoes
Sugar snap peas	Water chestnuts
*These vegetables are very high in vitamin A and should be eaten only once each day. Note: Dill pickles—limit to one serving per day due to high sodium content.	

Group Eight—Salad Greens

For both lunch and dinner, one cup of salad greens should be included in your meal. If desired, the vegetable exchange can be added to the salad greens.

SALAD GREENS	
Arugula	Mâche
Belgian endive	Mustard greens
Bibb lettuce	Napa cabbage
Boston lettuce	Romaine
Curly endive	Savoy cabbage
Dandelion greens	Spinach
Escarole	Swiss chard
Iceberg lettuce	Watercress
Note: Darker lettuce leaves are more nutrient rich and should be used more frequently.	

Group Nine—Fats

Select one item listed below per exchange—one serving is equal to five grams of fat. Use regular butter, margarine, mayonnaise, etc., and avoid diet, whipped, light, or low-calorie fats.

One Teaspoon Allowance		One Tablespoon Allowance
Butter	Olive oil	Commercial sugar-free salad dressing or vinaigrette
Hazelnut oil	Sesame oil	
Margarine	Vegetable oils	
Mayonnaise (sugar-free)	Walnut oil	

Group Ten—Condiments

Using nonfat dressings and condiments is optional, but they may be incorporated into your meal plan in small measure. You may also use one tablespoon per day of the following: horseradish, mustard, light soy sauce, steak sauce, Tabasco, or tamari.

MISCELLANEOUS CONDIMENTS	DRIED HERBS AND SPICES—UP TO 1 TSP. PER DAY	SAUCES—½ CUP PER DAY
Clear broth—no more than 1 cup/day (i.e., beef, poultry, fish, or vegetable)	Basil	Barbecue sauce
Equal or other sugar substitutes—no more than 6 packets/day	Cardamom	Picante sauce
Fat-free salad dressing—2 tablespoons per meal or up to ¼ cup per day	Cinnamon	Pizza sauce
Lemon juice—no more than 2 tablespoons/day	Curry	Salsa
Lemon wedges—no more than 6/day	Garlic	Spaghetti sauce
Vanilla (alcohol-free)—no more than 1 teaspoon/day	Nutmeg	Tomato sauce
	Oregano	V8 juice
	Tarragon	Vinegar

Note: Remember that sugar must be listed fifth or lower on the label of any condiment that you buy or use. If you use the full allotment in cooking, do not use it again at the table.

Group Eleven—Beverages

Hydration is crucial to any meal plan, most particularly through drinking water. However, you can add other sugar-free decaffeinated beverages to your plan, choosing two servings per day of any of the following, outside of water, which is unlimited.

- Sugar-free, caffeine-free sodas
- Decaf coffee
- Decaf or herbal tea
- Water

Group Twelve—Evening Snack

The evening snack should take place four to five hours after dinner using the dairy, cereal, and fruit requirements. When we are in a weight-loss program, our bodies are naturally trained to view this caloric reduction as starvation, a reaction that evolved over time from when food was scarce and any drop in intake meant malnourishment. In order to avoid this adaptation, we make a metabolic adjustment. This gives our bodies a boost before bed. Though we should try to eat an earlier dinner (between five and six p.m., so that our snack takes place between nine and ten p.m.), this snack can be eaten right before you go to bed. Because it adjusts the body's ability to metabolize the foods so it doesn't move into "conservation mode," it can be eaten late. This will also help folks who like to eat right before bed, or who wake up in the middle of the night to eat. It provides satiation without putting too much food in the stomach before sleep.

Mindful Eating

As living beings, we are blessed with earth's natural resources—its fruits, vegetables, grains, and meats—all given to us for our sustenance and survival. We can continue eating them mindlessly, grazing like cattle, devouring like wolves, or we can use the powerful minds with which we were also blessed to form a new relationship with those resources. Though we've been struggling with this relationship for centuries (the ancient philosopher Hippocrates even wrote, "If we could give every individual the right amount of nourishment and exercise, not too little and not too much, we would have found the safest way to health"), the time has come when that safest way must be followed.

But if you can't be honest about your food, or if you're playing with that magic math in your head, overscooping or underscooping your portions, you might not yet have surrendered. As long as you think that you can get away with it, or that you can manipulate the food plan set forth here, you are still holding on to that delusion of control.

As with any addiction, we need to make healthy choices in our life in order to avoid the substance or process that triggers the mental cravings of our dependency. I didn't eat a bite of sugar for the first eighteen years of my recovery, and then I got to thinking that maybe I could. I worked with a food sponsor to see whether it was possible, and I quickly discovered I wanted more. The addiction cycle was kicked off, and I was able to say, "Oops, this doesn't work." I cannot tell you what you are addicted to or what you need to quit, but I do suggest that you try your own experiment, and if you are not able to eat something without kicking off that craving (or suffering from its withdrawals), then you might consider abstaining from it.

By designing and preparing your meals in advance, you will discover what the great Saint Augustine once said: "Complete abstinence is easier than perfect moderation." As you look at the following empty chart, decide what your first week of sober and abstinent eating will look like, pulling from the lists of your favorite foods to put together a schedule of healthy meals, which include low-fat meats or meat substitutes, healthy starches, vegetables, fruits, fats, and dairy.

	MONDAY	TUESDAY	WEDNESDAY

Breakfast
2 oz. protein
1 oz. cereal
8 oz. low-fat
    milk or plain
    yogurt			

Lunch
3 oz. protein
    (women)
4 oz. protein
    (men)
½ cup starch
1 cup vegetables
1 cup salad
1 fat			

Dinner
3 oz. protein
    (women)
4 oz. protein
    (men)
½ cup starch
    (women)
1 cup starch
    (men)
1 cup vegetables
1 cup salad
1 fat			

Snack
8 oz. low-fat
    milk or plain
    yogurt
1 oz. cereal
1 fruit			

	THURSDAY	FRIDAY	SATURDAY	SUNDAY
Breakfast 2 oz. protein 1 oz. cereal 8 oz. low-fat milk or plain yogurt				
Lunch 3 oz. protein (women) 4 oz. protein (men) ½ cup starch 1 cup vegetables 1 cup salad 1 fat				
Dinner 3 oz. protein (women) 4 oz. protein (men) ½ cup starch (women) 1 cup starch (men) 1 cup vegetables 1 cup salad 1 fat				
Snack 8 oz. low-fat milk or plain yogurt 1 oz. cereal 1 fruit				

. . .

A diet is something you go *on,* and when you go *on* something that means you are going to go *off* it, too. Abstinence is not about dieting. It is not about doing everything perfectly, and throwing up your hands if you have to be a little flexible. If you go to a salad bar and the only starch available is white flour, say, saltines, then you eat the saltines. You don't bargain starches now for starches later, and you don't beat yourself up if you have to go a little off the path. You are through dieting. You are through believing that some miracle pill or unattainable weight is going to make you feel better, terrified that if you step off the path, you will never find a way to get back on.

A food plan is a strategy for healthy living, which becomes a working part of the mind and body, and an integral aspect of your recovery.

My dear friend Patty recently said that she knew she was recovered when she could still wear the same clothes from two years before. Prior to that time, she was 140 pounds overweight and had yo-yoed all over the scale, but then she came to Shades, committed to the meal plan, joined Overeaters Anonymous, and, after losing those 140 pounds, she has stayed at that healthy weight for the last two years.

Today I live life one day at a time, with that eye on forever. I know that as long as I am doing what is good, right, and honest for me in this moment, I can become present. Every pain is announced, every joy experienced, and hunger is but a tap on my shoulder for me to pay closer attention, reminding me that life does not take place in my troubled history nor in my unknown tomorrow. Mindfulness is now, and it is up to me to honor it.

PART SIX

Faith

I am not what happened to me, I am what I choose to become.

—CARL JUNG

THIRTEEN

The Road of Happy Destiny

*M*ost afternoons, once we are finished with our group sessions and staff meetings, working with families and new clients alike, I come home feeling like I just gave birth—exhausted and elated at once. Often I will get on the phone with friends, calling my sponsor, checking in with other women in Overeaters Anonymous, doing the work I need to do for my own recovery. One evening, however, I came home too tired to talk to anyone, instead settling in with RL to watch old movies, as we still enjoy doing. It was an early summer night, and though the sun might have set, a purple light spread across the sky. My phone rang and I saw it was Kim calling. I was about to invite her over for movie night when she told me that one of the clients had run away.

"Oh, Lord." I sighed. "Who is it this time?"

Kim replied, clearly disappointed, "Sharon."

Sharon had been to Shades before. The first time, she was one of our star clients, engaging actively in her recovery, focused on her inventories, and throwing herself into twelve-step work. Sharon was an athletic-looking blonde with tan skin and the vivacious personality of a cheer-leader. She had been married for a number of years to a supportive and wonderful man, Doug, and since they had never had children, their lives were devoted to each other. They shared hobbies, friends, and every aspect of their life, except for Sharon's bulimia, which she had kept secret from her husband for years. At first, she had attended only our six-day intensive program, but when she finished, Doug pleaded for her to stay for the six-week residential program. He was committed to seeing her recover, fearful of the desperation he had watched unfold at her disease's end, and so Sharon continued with us for six weeks, going home healthy.

A year later, Sharon came back a mess. The story she told us was not surprising. As much as Doug was supportive of her coming to treatment, when she got home he figured she was cured. He didn't understand why she needed to go to meetings or get together with her sponsor, expecting her to participate in their relationship as before—going waterskiing, snowboarding, traveling with friends, and socializing every weekend. He told her she didn't need the meetings, and would get irritated when she went.

As much as he wanted to see her healthy, he figured that was what Shades was for. He didn't respect or understand that recovery is a lifetime commitment. Instead of fighting him on it, Sharon stopped attending Anorexics and Bulimics Anonymous. Sadly, it didn't take long for her to be right back in her disease, resuming the laxatives and the self-hatred that are endemic to the binge-purge cycle. Once again, Doug was in the dark—until the morning Sharon collapsed in the bathroom, her house of lies falling down around her.

One of the most difficult and necessary parts of recovery comes in the renegotiation of our lives, forcing us to confront reality without our old defense mechanisms to protect us. We will soon discover that our old ways of doing things simply don't work any longer, as the road gets narrower, demanding that we change our behaviors in order to protect our abstinence.

As for Sharon, she returned to Shades without the enthusiasm that she had brought with her before. She wasn't here because of Doug, trying to please him and save their relationship through treatment. This time around, when Sharon's spouse came for Family Week, we didn't focus on Doug's commitment to Sharon's health, but rather on Sharon's surrender.

Doug sat in the small room where we meet with families one-on-one. Also athletic and attractive, he looked like the star athlete next to Sharon's cheerleader. Together, they made the "perfect couple"—no one knowing the sickness that lived in their home because they had created such a handsome illusion to protect it. Sharon's parents were also there, sympathetic to this work, if a bit confused, but Doug was bewildered. He wasn't addicted to anything, was able to drink and eat in normal moderation. Enjoying a good meal, he could appreciate fine dining and pastries as much as a burger and fries; he didn't experience the effects that Sharon did.

He held her hand and asked, "Baby, it's just that we've been here before; how are we here again?"

She looked down, unable to answer until I began to explain. "Sharon, you don't need to beat yourself up for this. You didn't screw up the first time; it's just that you also didn't surrender. Compliance is a half surrender—it is there to prove that we are normal, that folks don't need to worry about us. There was a great doctor who once did a lot of work on addiction, Dr. Harry Tiebout, who said that compliance 'means agreeing, going along with, but in no way implies enthusiastic, wholehearted assent and approval.'"

"But she was so excited," Doug argued. "She was enthusiastic!"

"It's not about acting enthusiastic—I don't trust anyone who comes to treatment thrilled. No one wants to be in treatment, Doug. We don't want to be told what to do, or that what we've been doing all along is wrong, but that deep, wholehearted consent is a different enthusiasm. Sharon, the question is: Do you want to be here?"

Sharon didn't reply. Later that day, she ran off.

That evening, after receiving the call about Sharon, I picked Kim up at the main administrative building at Shades in the golf cart I frequently drive around our property. We decided to go up one of the old country roads that lead out of the center, thinking that if Sharon went walking, she might have headed that way. As we passed the neighbors' houses, the long wheat-colored fields of west Texas, and even those old cows up the road, I couldn't help but remember when I, too, had run from treatment.

For many addicts, reality is hell. They have been avoiding it their whole lives, growing up in households where the truth was too much to bear, or they were too sensitive to bear it. Addicts have to find a way out, and through food, love, shopping, they do, until the addiction stops working. And then they start to heal, and the pain returns. That reality begins to sink in, and they are so raw, so wholly unprepared for it, they just want to stop. Suddenly their lives before don't look so bad, and they think they can figure it out on their own, but if they could, they wouldn't need to buy the books or go on the diets or end up at a place like Shades.

I looked over at Kim, and I remembered how, on my third day at treatment, I received the call that Kim had tried to kill herself. She was severely anorexic, and would soon be joining me at that facility in Los Angeles. As heartbreaking as it is to recall, I had run away because I didn't want Kim to come. I couldn't imagine bearing the grief of seeing that broken child without my "medicine." Food had always been my way to escape reality, and now I was being asked to face that reality without my primary source of comfort. How was I, her mother, going to walk through the guilt and shame and fear of her near death? Instead,

I walked out into the dangerous Los Angeles neighborhood where our treatment center was located, heading down the street in the shorts, T-shirt, and flip-flops they had us wear. I was crying and swearing, and if anyone had passed me, they would have assumed I was an indigent.

I got to the end of that block, and I knew that I couldn't keep running away; I couldn't run from me, from Kim, my disease, or the feelings that in that moment seemed far too hard to accept. Sirens blared, helicopters flew overhead, there was commotion all around me, and then as though from another voice, I remembered the prescription one of AA's cofounders wrote for recovery early on in that organization's history. He had suggested that as long as we always remember to "trust God, clean house, help others," healing could be ours.

I watched as Kim scanned the horizon looking for Sharon, and felt utterly blessed that both of us had stopped running.

Faith Employed

Over the last twenty-five years, I have found that the miracle of living does not come in life itself but in how we choose to live it. For decades I believed in the illusion of control. I thought that if I had a vise grip on life, everything would go according to my plans, but after nearly strangling my relationships—and myself—to death, I finally had to concede that I could control very little in this world. I could not control my husband's drinking, my children's choices, or even my own outcomes. When I finally turned that illusion back over to the God of my understanding, I loosened my hands and allowed life to proceed. Did that mean that it went exactly how I wanted it go? Certainly not. But what it did mean was that I could better embrace life, no longer needing to deny my emotions or wrest everything from everyone; I could just be still and know it was in God's hands.

This didn't happen overnight, and I didn't do it on my own. Because the other side of letting go was realizing that I did have some control—and that was over my own behaviors. When I chose to ask for help, I received it. I started doing what was right in front of me rather than what was way beyond me. I started moving forward, my faith increasing as I went.

Kim and I had approached the railroad tracks that run from Abilene through Buffalo Gap when Kim saw a small figure in the distance, walking along the railroad ties.

"Well, hell," I said, turning onto the tracks.

Kim laughed. "Mother, we're gonna scare the life out of her, coming down like this."

"I think it's about time she dealt with a little fear."

As we moved down the tracks, Sharon heard us approach. She turned around, wide-eyed that we had found her.

Kim hopped out of the golf cart. "Evening. What are you doing up here?"

Sharon shrugged. "I just wanted to go for a walk, okay? Where I am going to go, anyway? It's like you guys chose to be out here so none of us could escape."

I joined them. "Well, we didn't think about it at the time, but it has helped. When I ran away from treatment, I was too terrified of the neighborhood we were in to go far . . . and I thank God every day for that."

Kim countered, "I've broken out of almost every treatment I've been in, including the one they sent me to with Mother. Can you imagine being in treatment with your own mother?"

Sharon laughed. "Oh, God, how do you people work together?"

I looked at Kim and smiled. "It's called a miracle, Sharon. All three of us standing here, watching the night approach, and yes, Kim's and my relationship included, this is all a miracle. For me, once I was able to start living life step by step, one day at a time, I began to realize that faith wasn't about life looking how I wanted or expected it to look; faith was about my accepting life as it is, surrendering to all the things over which I had little or no control."

There is a beautiful passage in the classic text *Alcoholics Anonymous*: "Acceptance is the answer to *all* my problems today. When I am disturbed, it is because I find some person, place, thing, or situation—some fact of my life—unacceptable to me, and I can find no serenity until I accept that person, place, thing, or situation as being exactly the way it is supposed to be at this moment. Nothing, absolutely nothing happens in God's world by mistake."

Sharon stood there, wearing a T-shirt, shorts, and flip-flops, and I felt like we were back in 1985, when I also didn't know how to accept the addiction that was then so evident.

Finally Sharon began to share, opening up for the first time since she had returned to Shades. "I've been in control my whole life. That's why I haven't even wanted kids. You know Doug does; he would love them, but I like being in charge of my life. The last time when I got home, I thought that I could do it by myself, learn what you all had taught me, and then I would get better. I wouldn't need help carrying it out."

Kim replied in that slow Texas drawl she inherited from RL. "I get it. Girl, I spent years trying to do it on my own, by myself, and finally I had to hit my knees, saying, 'This way of life doesn't work for me anymore. I don't like who I am and who I have become. I want to be different, and I want to feel different. Someone please help me.' That illusion of control had to be surrendered in order for help to come."

Miraculously, help came for both Kim and me. It came in the form of the people who saved my life, and the folks who saved Kim's. And as we have continued along the road of recovery, it has come in every relationship we have uncovered, discovered, and discarded—with our-selves, with others, and with God. We stopped pretending that every-thing was perfect, that we were so strong and stoic, that nothing could get through our "boundaries" when really everything did.

I explained, "Being healthy in recovery means being able to stand tall and be autonomous with the God of your understanding. It is about having a God you trust, and recognizing that He, She, It, whatever has been there all along, but you need to open yourself to other people in order to see that."

My first gods, outside of Snoopy, were all the people I met in recov-ery: women like my best friend, Pat, and Dr. Hollis, and later Pia Mel-lody and my other wonderful friends. They were my higher power when I didn't know where else to find God, and today, in many ways, they still are. God reveals Himself in various ways, often through the angels that are sent into our lives, helping us to see God everywhere. His messages become clear, and as Kim, Sharon, and I stood there, we saw one before our eyes, flitting through the evening sky.

Kim saw the cardinal first, pointing it out to Sharon and me as it landed in a nearby tree, staring at these three crazy ladies hanging out on the railroad tracks. Kim told us, "The cardinal in Native American understanding represents change. Every time you see one, you can be sure that very big transformations, those crossroads in your life, are about to emerge."

Sharon smiled. "Is that what you call a miracle?"

Sometimes we don't have to look very far for miracles. Every minute you go without practicing your addiction is a miracle, and every family who reunites shares in the same joy. On a daily basis, I watch families reunite and relationships heal. However, it's a miracle that takes a lot of work. We have to relearn how to be in relationships with others, and then, through those relationships, we begin to see God everywhere.

Time Takes Time

It was Theo's last day at Shades. After ten months, he had lost more than ninety pounds, dropping from 530 to 426. Having started out in our six-week residential program, he had continued on in our transition housing, ultimately moving into one of the halfway houses on our property. Like many folks who suffer from morbid obesity, he came in hoping that treatment would immediately remove the weight, taking only months for him to go from an absolutely unmanageable size to something entirely unrealistic. His whole life he had spent in hiding, refusing to take responsibility for his behaviors, blaming his parents (divorced), his upbringing (isolated), and his access to food (plentiful) for his weight. But as he continued in recovery, he realized that he wasn't just losing weight; he was learning, slowly but surely, how to live.

Time takes time. Just as with Theo's weight loss, nothing happens overnight. We are building and developing new habits so that they become embedded in our behavior. They're second nature, whereas before our first nature was to eat and ignore, masking our true selves in a swath of food.

I walked up to the dining hall as dinner was about to begin and saw Theo sitting outside on the porch, looking out across the campus.

"You ready to leave?" I asked.

His fear was apparent. "I don't know. I keep wondering whether I can make it out there. I know I have the support, but what if I screw up?"

"You know, it's a nasty misconception that we have to go to the bottom of the pit just because of one slip. Instead of seeing relapse—if, God forbid, that happens—as the end, you can view it as a warning. But more than that, there is work you can do to see it coming."

Your food plan is an amazing barometer. When folks relapse with food, it's never about the food; it's always about something going on in their lives. As you go forth, whenever you start hungering for more than is in your plan, all you need to do is sit down, breathe deep, and do three simple things:

1. Ask for God to help remove the mental obsession. The Serenity Prayer is a powerful and easy pause to remember where you are powerless and where you can be courageous, seeking wisdom in both.
2. Look to what you're feeling in that moment, and identify whether it's anger, pain, fear, loneliness, shame, guilt, or joy. How can you process that emotion, embracing it as a gift?
3. Find someone to call who will understand your plight—a friend, your food sponsor, someone who might also need help—and let him or her in on what you are thinking about eating, and why.

I sat down next to Theo. "You don't have to go all the way back into your disease to see that something's foul, Theo. If you start craving more fats or want to add starches to your plan, you know to stop yourself and take an inventory. We clean house, and then we are able to see what is triggering that need, provoking that temptation for relapse. There is no end to recovery. Even if we do fall off our meal plan, Overeaters Anonymous meetings and the people within it don't disappear in our absence. They are always there, waiting for us with loving arms."

We need to take relapse seriously, but we don't need to treat it like it's the end of the world. Time takes time, and the more patient and steady we become, the farther along we find ourselves, until one day relapse fails to beckon, and recovery becomes our permanent home.

The Shades of Hope Miracle

The most beautiful part of healing is that you don't have to do it alone. There are other people who will help you along the way—other recovering people who have learned that in order to keep the gift of abstinence, they had to be willing to open themselves up to others. They had to get involved with like kinds so that they could finally get out of their own heads and learn to share their experience, strength, and hope with someone else. All my life I had been terrified of other people. Though professionally, I knew how to counsel folks and ask them the right questions, if you wanted me to share anything of myself, forget it. As a child I had few friends, alienated by my peers because of my weight and my home life. Today, my world is filled with friendship, built on those relationships I discovered in recovery. As I reached out for help, or as someone reached out to me, we connected in ways that few spirits do: offering the raw and vulnerable parts of ourselves as the foundation of friendship. We do not respond to the question, "How are you?" with, "Fine." We open our hearts willingly, allowing our fears to come out, crying as our relationships with our husbands, wives, and friends ebb and flow. Together, we dream of the choices we can make to live better, and then we offer one another the guidance and support to see those dreams realized.

Food had been Theo's companion for decades, until he came to Shades and began to meet others who shared his experience. He described:

> Initially, fellowship was so hard for me. I used to stutter when I talked to people. But I am able to have healthy relationships today, and I've been able to see how important they are for my recovery. I started working with other people, new men who came to Shades, and I've seen they are just like me, and I love them for it. When I am able to have close relationships I don't need my eating disorder.

When I am working with someone else, I am not thinking about me, about my needs or even my hunger. Today I no longer live in a dark and damp basement; I live in a glass house. I am—whether good, bad, or otherwise—infamously honest, able to shine that bright light of reflection on my own life as well as someone else's. I don't need to wear that clown's mask anymore. Even today, when I do something that doesn't feel good, right, or honest, either forgetting to eat the scheduled cereal on my meal plan in the morning, or treating someone in a way of which I am not proud, I open that big mouth I am so famous for and I tell on myself to someone else. And in doing so, I invite that other person to be honest as well.

That is why a major tenet of the twelve-step program is sponsorship. A sponsor is a person who has worked the twelve steps, and who can take you through the same, offering what was so freely given to him or her. It is suggested that you check in with a sponsor every day and let her know how you're doing, what you're eating, and whether there are any issues that need to be addressed. It is a gift to both the sponsor and the sponsee. It allows the sponsee a safe place to be himself or herself. And it presents the sponsor with an opportunity each day to step out of her head, her worries, fantasies, and self-obsession, and help someone who shares her disease.

One of the greatest joys of working in treatment is getting to see that same gift blossom in the lives of our clients. It is the Shades of Hope miracle. Folks who were either killing themselves or refusing to live come alive, reaching out, sponsoring other men and women. And as they watch someone else begin to thrive, they are finally able to see it in themselves. That's how recovery happens—it is all about getting with other like kinds. Clients might be here only two weeks, but then they're telling someone else their story, getting honest in ways they never have before, and they begin to grow like flowers reaching for the light.

The Family Forward

Kim, Sharon, and I stood on that railroad track for quite some time that night. We all shared our experiences of what it was like to be addicted to food, what happened to force us to surrender and seek recovery, and what our lives and families have been like now that we live in healing.

Sharon worried. "What if I change? What if Doug doesn't love the new me?"

"Did he come here for Family Week?" I asked, to which Sharon nodded yes. "Sharon, Doug wants the healthiest version of you; it is why he's been so supportive. But you also have to see that this is where faith comes in. As you begin to heal, Doug will also get the chance to participate in healing. If he wants to do that, which it seems he does, then you will both change. The healthier we get, the more we want to be with a healthy person, and yes, you might find yourselves on separate paths at first, but then you'll realize that you're going in the same direction. When we stand alone, we can stand together. Otherwise, you're just two sick people leaning up against each other, until someone finally falls, bringing the whole thing down."

Sharon looked away. "I've been leaning against Doug our whole marriage."

"And he's used to that; it's why your going to meetings was scary for him."

Doug had always been Sharon's support network, but Doug didn't have an eating disorder. He didn't understand the thoughts and feelings that Sharon was contending with, seeing her recovery as a six-week deal rather than a lifetime commitment. On her second trip to Shades, Sharon stayed for three months. Though it was tough on Doug, he knew that it was a matter of life or death, realizing that this time Sharon was committed to her recovery plan. She had surrendered, and he needed to surrender, too.

This time, when Sharon returned home, she threw herself into Anorexics and Bulimics Anonymous. Though it was hard at first for their relationship, Sharon's new commitment to her health gave Doug the chance to create some healthy outlets as well. He got more involved in hobbies he was always interested in, creating fellowship with other men, rather than always expecting Sharon to be his company. After Sharon was abstinent from bulimia for over a year, she and Doug decided that they wanted to grow their family, working on getting pregnant for the first time in their relationship. Kim and I were not surprised, remembering back to that night when we all finally headed home. Sharon sat next to me in the cart, Kim riding in the back as Sharon told us, "I always thought I was too sick to bring someone else into this world. They would have this mother who didn't know how to be healthy, how to be there for anyone but herself and her disease. I didn't think things could ever change, that change was possible, but it is, isn't it?"

I looked at my daughter, who sat peacefully in the back, a completely different woman from the depressed and feral child I had once tried to raise. I winked. "It's possible for anyone, anywhere, at any time; you just have to say, 'I'll take it.'"

My Hope for You

As I drove us all back to Shades of Hope, we passed the sign that sits in front of the main building. When we were first opening our facility, we struggled and struggled with a name. I was so frustrated; I thought we would end up calling it McCarty Oil, like our other family business. The renovations were almost complete, and RL was getting tired of my inability to stick a sign out front explaining what the heck this was all for. I invited a close friend and one of Shades' early business partners, Carmen, to come and see the property, proud of what we were creating, even if it didn't have a name.

She brought along her son Eric Stackhouse, who was fourteen years old at the time and who happened to be an incredible artist, carrying along with him a sketch pad. In the middle of the property stood a large and imposing oak, its branches swept over our facility like loving arms, light filtered through its leaves creating shadow and shade across the yard. It was majestic, and Eric was immediately engrossed. He sat down to sketch the tree while his mother and I walked around the grounds. When we returned, he was already finished. He had drawn the tree to perfection, and under it had written, "Shades of Hope."

If we are willing to listen, God will always speak to us. And that is what recovery offers—it gives us all shades of hope. For some, it might be the hope that they can let go of their childhood traumas; for others, it might be the hope that they can break their dependency on food; and for yet others, they might simply hope to love themselves. They are tired of addiction, convinced that's not what they have, but ultimately becoming grateful that their problem is actually as simple and uncomplicated as that. Whether the substance is food, drugs, nicotine, or alcohol, or the process is shopping, sex, gambling, work, or codependence, we get something from the outside that helps us to feel better on the inside, and we feel worse when we do not have it.

My greatest hope is that you will finish this book, realizing that the tools you learned when you were young (whether it was overeating, looking perfect, keeping quiet, or some other behavior) are no longer assets but liabilities. It is time to pick up a new set of tools—ones that will allow you to pass through life on the easy wings of faith and not with the desperate need of dependency.

When Kim finally returned to Buffalo Gap, sober, healthy, and abstinent, we had to learn how to build a new relationship. It wasn't easy. And once we started to work together, we had to create a whole new dance. Our old relationship would not have served us or anyone at Shades of Hope. And so we began to work toward healing. I stopped seeing her as the scapegoat, and she stopped seeing me as the evil witch who had done her wrong. We set aside our old ideas, and we found a whole new experience. After we dropped Sharon off, I drove Kim back to the house in which she now lives in Buffalo Gap. When Kim was young, the building was a local church, where she would often run and pray, hiding out from the mayhem that was our family. Today that church is her home; her living room is the space where pews once sat, and, ironically enough, the altar is now her kitchen. I pulled up and looked over, my beautiful daughter having fallen asleep on our drive, and tears filled my eyes with the miracle that is healing. She woke up and kissed me on the cheek, squeezing my hand, and said the words that at one point were unutterable between us: "I love you, Mama." She got out and walked into the house, and my heart just broke with joy. That is the gift of recovery: to free us enough from ourselves that we may finally be in true and powerful relationship with others.

I drove back through Buffalo Gap that evening, the stars hanging like lightbulbs, breathing in the warm night air, my arms and thighs and belly finally befitting the woman inside, and that once-broken spirit surged with light. From my deepest, most powerful place, I was fulfilled.

As you stand at your own crossroads, I can only hope that you allow your higher power to illuminate the adventure before you, casting away your shadows so that you may finally participate in healing. If you are willing to surrender to the process, to try something new and fun and wholly terrifying, the journey will be yours for the taking. You will discover that divine self within, which has been held in God's grace, and is now yours to nourish.

Appendix

Recovery is about reclaiming the life you always sought, but feared to achieve. Since my first days in a twelve-step program, I recognized that they offered more than just a solution to my codependence, my overeating, or my bulimia; they were handing us the tools of how to live in and process an unpredictable and at times quite painful world. If you are now ready to surrender, and not just comply with the world around you, you will be able to walk into recovery knowing that you are about to receive a second chance at this life, one free from addiction. You will be released from the past and no longer threatened by the unknown tomorrow. God is in the present, and you are sure to find that higher power of your understanding amid the fellowship and wisdom of the twelve steps and those they have healed.

If you are ready to heal your issues with food, Overeaters Anonymous, Anorexics and Bulimics Anonymous, *and* Food Addicts in Recovery all offer incredible recovery resources from food addiction and eating disorders. Another source of available help is ACORN Food Dependency Recovery Services' ACORN Primary Intensive, which offers comprehensive services for those suffering with food addiction. For specialists desiring in-depth training on how to deal with the mental, emotional, and spiritual issues relating to food addiction, the Food Addiction Institute's three-year training program is a wonderful option for professionals.

- Overeaters Anonymous—www.oa.org; 505-891-2664
- Anorexics and Bulimics Anonymous—www.aba12steps.org; 780-318-6355
- Food Addicts in Recovery—www.foodaddicts.org; 781-932-6300
- ACORN Food Dependency Recovery Services—www.foodaddiction .com; 941-378-2122
- Food Addiction Institute—www.foodaddictioninstitute.org; 941-747-1972

For your dependency on shopping or spending, Debtors Anonymous can teach you how to live abundantly and within your means. Clutterers Anonymous can help with excessive hoarding, and Gamblers Anonymous has proven to be very successful with those facing gambling addiction.

- Debtors Anonymous—www.debtorsanonymous.org; 800-421-2383
- Clutterers Anonymous—www.sites.google.com/site/clutterersanony mous; 310-281-6064
- Gamblers Anonymous—www.gamblersanonymous.org; 213-386-8789

If you fear you are having issues managing or maintaining a healthy sex life, Sex and Love Anonymous as well as Sex Addicts Anonymous are incredibly powerful programs. Also, if you have experienced sexual trauma or abuse, Survivors of Incest Anonymous is a safe and important start to healing the abused child within.

- Sex and Love Addicts Anonymous—www.slaafws.org; 210-828-7900
- Sex Addicts Anonymous—www.saa-recovery.org; 800-477-8191
- Survivors of Incest Anonymous—www.siawso.org; 410-893-3322

In order to deal with the addictions others in your family have or have had, Al-Anon and Alateen are important groups for anyone who has suffered the consequences of another person's addiction. Whether you are tired of losing yourself in others or refusing to engage in emotional partnerships, Codependents Anonymous will show you how to stand on your own and yet still be in a relationship. And for those who are in partnership with another recovering adult, Recovering Couples Anonymous can help you to heal and grow together.

- Al-Anon—www.al-anon.org; 888-425-2666
- Alateen—www.al-anon.alateen.org; 757-563-1600
- Codependents Anonymous—www.coda.org; 888-444-2359
- Recovering Couples Anonymous—www.recovering-couples.org; 877-663-2317

And finally, if you are suffering from chemical dependency, there are programs for any addiction you might be struggling with: Alcoholics Anonymous for alcoholism, Narcotics Anonymous for prescription medication and other narcotic drugs, Nicotine Anonymous, and more.

- Alcoholics Anonymous—www.aa.org; 714-556-4555
- Narcotics Anonymous—www.na.org; 800-477-6291
- Nicotine Anonymous—www.nicotine-anonymous.org; 877-879-6422
- Cocaine Anonymous—www.ca.org; 310-559-5833
- Crystal Meth Anonymous—www.crystalmeth.org; 213-488-4455

There are meetings in nearly every city, and in them you will find people who are tired of dwelling in their problems and who seek to live in solutions. When our clients leave Shades, we recommend they try six different meetings in every program to which they relate. If you are overeating, then try six different Overeaters Anonymous meetings, and though you may not like every one of them, keep an open mind until you find the one where you feel at home. You are worth six hours in order to find the program and place that can finally help you to live the divine and purposeful life you have always deserved. As my sponsor, Pat, says, "You already are what you've always wanted to be."

Acknowledgments

The making of this book has been a journey, and it has taken many people to bring it into reality. First and foremost, the credit goes to my youngest daughter, Kristi McCarty. Kristi has encouraged and supported me for years to tell my story in writing, and has done much of the footwork to bring this project into reality. This book would not exist without her, nor would our wonderful treatment center, Shades of Hope, that has been successfully managed and realized through Kristi's hard work and dedication. Kristi—I love and appreciate you!

Every once in a while, God puts someone in our lives who wiggles their way into our hearts and stays there permanently. God put that love in my heart for my adopted granddaughter, Ashley Judd. It is as if we have known each other forever, proving to me yet again that love is the most powerful force in the world.

Thanks to Ashley, I have been so fortunate to work with Trena Keating, our talented and experienced literary agent, who has lent both her wisdom and sound advice to this work.

Through Trena, we met our incredible publisher and editor, Amy Einhorn. On our trip to New York to consult with prospective publishers, Amy was the first one Kristi and I met. With her beautiful warm smile and her intense interest in what I had to say, I knew Amy was the one. Kristi and I have been business partners for years, and sometimes when we have a big decision ahead of us, we will write down our first choice and then compare notes. Kristi and I had both written Amy's name. It was a very wise decision.

God put another angel in my life along the way to help give structure to my thoughts and beliefs. Kristen McGuiness has worked diligently on this book and brings her own experience in addiction and recovery to the table. We speak the same language.

I want to thank my parents, Thad and Neva Johnson. With all their dysfunction and sickness, they somehow gave me the courage to change the cycle of addiction that is passed down from generation to generation. I knew from a very early age that I was going to break the cycle, and by God's grace and with the help of many angels, the cycle has been broken. I choose to believe my parents would have been proud of me.

Many thanks to my sweetheart, Mr. Mac. We've been through heaven and hell together and he still remains my best supporter. RL has believed in me for almost forty-nine years. Without his emotional support—and financial, too—there would be no Shades of Hope. Thank you, honey.

To my middle daughter, Kimberly June—thank you for teaching me one of the great lessons of recovery. Starting at a young age, Kim started acting out the dysfunctions of her parents, becoming the one to get our family help. Today she is one of my best friends and one of the most talented therapists I know. The more pain we suffer and recover from, the more we have to give to others.

Many thanks to my most precious oldest daughter, Karen. She always challenges me to reach a higher level. She is one of the most intelligent women I know—always has been, always will be. Karen has a loving and caring soul, and we are so grateful she has made her way to Shades of Hope to work with our clients. It has been quite an amazing journey, and it's not over.

My appreciation goes to my son, Kelly, who in his own quiet way believes in me and the work we do at Shades. He has become a very successful businessman and has on more than one occasion helped me financially to keep the dream alive. I thank you, son.

ACKNOWLEDGMENTS

God has put beloved women in my life to teach me and grow with me. The first of these is my beloved friend and spiritual adviser Pat Huber. She has played many roles in our family, primarily the grandmother my children never had. She has attended every birthday, funeral, graduation, dance, and prom, and just keeps showing up for us all. Pat taught me what love is by loving me unconditionally. She shows me God in action, and she's also my best dancing partner.

When I think of my friend Cindy Lu Henson, my heart skips a beat. In our relationship she has had many faces—from client to friend to one of the most important people in my life. Cindy has a way of telling me about myself while still loving me. We've taken many trips together, including one to New Zealand, where she literally saved my life. For that and much more, I will always be grateful.

Dr. Kathy Easterling has given me the sister relationship I never had before—she is my sister of choice. Kathy has taught me never to burn bridges and that everyone is due second and third chances.

To my precious grandchildren—Natalie, Kaitlyn, Kaylie, Kyle, and Spencer B—you have delighted me in ways that are hard to describe. A love for a grandchild goes deeper than any love I've ever experienced. Although I don't get to see the older ones as much, they are in my prayers daily. Spencer B, the light of my life, has given me the wonderful opportunity to watch him grow and change on a daily basis. He has taught me how to play and laugh at myself.

My appreciation to the staff at Shades of Hope. Through the years they have made contributions toward making my dreams a reality. I could never have done this without them. My extreme thanks to Cam Balcomb, our executive director, beloved partner to my daughter Kristi, and "Momcee" to my sweet grandson Spencer B.

In 1985, through a series of divine interventions, I found myself inside a treatment center in Los Angeles. God put Judi Hollis, the director of the center, in my life. She is one of my many angels, and she changed me forever. Thanks, Jude!

Many thanks to my colleagues in the field who have entrusted me enough to refer clients to us—you know who you are. I am truly honored to have had the opportunity to work with some of the pioneers in the field of addiction, eating disorders, trauma, codependency, and others. Thank you for paving the way.

Last but certainly not least, thank you to the clients I have been privileged to work with. Our clients have taught me far more than I have ever taught them. To recovering folks everywhere, thank you for keeping the doors open and always welcoming me into the rooms that have saved my life. This journey of mine has been a life of uncovering, discovering, and discarding. If I can recover, anyone on the face of the earth can. If only you are willing to take a few simple steps each day, to follow a few simple directions, you, too, may look forward to "trudging the road of happy destiny."

About the Author

As the co-founder, CEO, and co-owner of Shades of Hope Treatment Center, Tennie McCarty brings over thirty years of combined professional and personal insight to the treatment of compulsive overeating, bulimia, anorexia, and other addictive disorders. She was the first program director at Serenity House in Abilene, Texas, a position she held for nine years, and is a licensed counselor in chemical dependency, alcohol and drug addiction, and eating disorders. She is also a certified addictions specialist.

In 1987, Tennie saw the need for an all-addiction treatment program. She and a partner founded Shades of Hope that year as a treatment center to address multiple addictions including eating disorders, alcoholism, chemical dependency, sexual addiction, self-injury histories, and codependency. Tennie speaks several times each year to professional groups throughout the country, including being asked to address Kentucky's American Medical Association in 2008.

In recovery herself and the mother of a recovering anorexic, Tennie has a unique insight into the nature of disordered eating, as featured on the Oprah Winfrey Network's program *Addicted to Food*. In addition, she has appeared on *The Ruby Show* for the Style Network, A&E's *Intervention*, *The Dr. Oz Show*, *The Joy Behar Show*, *Weekend Today* with Brad Lamm, and others. Tennie and her husband live in Buffalo Gap, Texas, home of Shades of Hope, where they are the parents to four grown children and grandparents to many.